CULTURAL LOCATIONS
OF DISABILITY

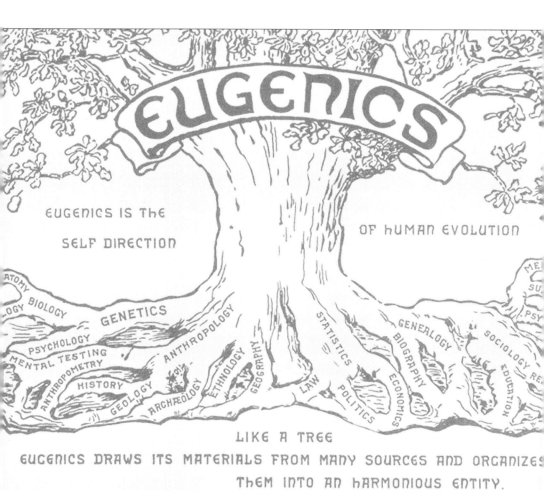

SHARON L. SNYDER
AND
DAVID T. MITCHELL

CULTURAL
LOCATIONS
OF
DISABILITY

THE UNIVERSITY OF
CHICAGO PRESS

CHICAGO AND LONDON

Sharon L. Snyder and David T. Mitchell are faculty in the
Department of Disability and Human Development at the University
of Illinois at Chicago. They are the authors of *Narrative Prosthesis:
Disability and the Dependencies of Discourse*, and editors of
The Body and Physical Difference: Discourses of Disability; *Eugenics
in America, 1848–1945: A History of Disability in Primary Sources*; and
The Encyclopedia of Disability.

The University of Chicago Press, Chicago 60637

The University of Chicago Press, Ltd., London

© 2006 by The University of Chicago

All rights reserved. Published 2006

Printed in the United States of America

15 14 13 12 11 10 09 08 07 06   1 2 3 4 5

ISBN: 0-226-76731-0 (cloth)

ISBN: 0-226-76732-9 (paper)

Library of Congress Cataloging-in-Publication Data

Snyder, Sharon L., 1963–

Cultural locations of disability /
Sharon L. Snyder and David T. Mitchell.

p. cm.

Includes bibliographical references and index.

ISBN: 0-226-76731-0 (cloth : alk. paper)—

ISBN: 0-226-76732-9 (pbk. : alk. paper)

1. Sociology of disability. 2. People with disabilities—
Social conditions. 3. People with disabilities—
Government policy. 4. People with disabilities in
motion pictures. I. Mitchell, David T., 1962– II. Title.

HV1568.S69 2006

305.9'08—dc22

2005020957

♾The paper used in this publication meets
the minimum requirements of the American
National Standard for Information
Sciences—Permanence of Paper
for Printed Library Materials,
ANSI Z39.48–1992.

(Anti-)Dedication
To the five Supreme Court justices in
the *Garrett v. State of Alabama* case who
claimed that no documented history exists
of systemic discrimination against
people with disabilities

DEDICATION
To those who lived this history
and who continue to negotiate
its aftershocks

CONTENTS

We cannot remember when the exact idea for this book came into being. In part it might have been during the development of essays about various confining locations that restrain disabled people and prevent them from meaningful participation. Or, perhaps, the idea of locations of culture came while we sifted through primary source materials written during the U.S. eugenics period, which were housed in David Braddock's archive on developmental disability at the University of Illinois at Chicago. Before we undertook that research, the concept of eugenics as a key shaper of disability policy, thought, and practice in the twentieth century was shaky at best. Within an otherwise disastrous historical legacy of the cultural policing of the country's "genetic stock," eugenics seemed somehow marginal and certainly antiquated as a meaningful influence on the cultural imagination about disability. Like many others, we thought of eugenics as a distant memory or ideology that had collapsed under the weight of its own inertia, incoherence, and ill-fated prophecies. Eugenics seemed remote, like witch hunting or public flogging—violent performances upon the bodies of those deemed unacceptable.

But the more deeply we delved into the body of literature on eugenics, the more it appeared to provide opportunities for imagining today's disability practices. As eugenics came increasingly to delineate a concept of substandard labor capacities—then identified largely through classifications such as idiocy, feeblemindedness, or subnormalcy—it started to give the category of disability a coherence that it hadn't quite had for us prior to our investigation into this literature. Eugenic thought, it seemed, had played a crucial role in defining a distinctive U.S. version of deviance that allowed physical, sensory, and cognitive differences to shadow each other—as if one could not be called into being without the others. These concepts of unbridgeable, biologically based otherness played host to myriad cultural definitions. As the philosopher of modernity Zygmunt Bauman argues, the Holocaust was not an aberration of modernity but rather its inevitable product. In a similar manner we began to understand that the categorization of disability as pathological deviance was not an excursion from normalcy but rather its ultimate product. Many in disability studies—from Lennard Davis to Rosemarie Garland Thomson to Henri-Jacques Stiker—had argued various versions of this point, but eugenics gave the theory a substance that it had never quite achieved before in our minds. Eugenics, as an influential hegemonic formation, increasingly struck us as not "over." Instead it lurked like a social phantasm just below the surface, determining the standards, manner, and parameters of our cultural, political, and intellectual debate about embodied differences.

Consequently, it seemed appropriate to inquire more closely into the nature of eugenic thought and its continuing reverberations in the lives of disabled people. We mean the phrase "cultural locations of disability" to evoke sites of violence, restriction, confinement, and absence of liberty for people with disabilities. In many ways this book hails a new form of cultural onslaught galvanized by new media environments: scientific, medical, popular, and technical writings on disability in the eugenics and post-eugenics period all collude together in constituting a bereft subject as disabled—as properly the subject for eugenic care, control, rehabilitation, evaluation, roundup, exclusion, and social erasure. (We use the term *bereft* in the sense of lacking capacity, integralness, aesthetic symmetry, competitive labor power, racial homogeneity, appropriate class boundaries, and assimilationist promise.) In part 1 we sample the key ideas extant in U.S.—and ultimately European—eugenics. The chapters in this opening section explore a minefield of conflicting notions while providing a meta-critical overview of basic tenets in the science of defective heredity and a bare-bones outline of the science of eugenics. The remaining two parts of the work trace some of the ramifications of these late-nineteenth- and early twentieth-century beliefs about disabilities, in order not simply to establish later twentieth-century forms of disability control as identical with those of this earlier period, but rather to assess to what extent the cultural imaginary of disability is still influenced by early eugenic thought. In other words, we seek to identify the degree to which eugenics subjects can be said to have metamorphosed into what we recognize today as "disability." All of this leads to a concluding contemplation of the institutionalization of disability studies in today's academy. Eugenics ideology survives in the willingness of today's disability research industries to treat the time and bodies of disabled persons as if they are inexhaustible. At-large, poorer populations and confined groups serve as lab rats for investigative projects. How do we rethink the ethics of research to allow disabled persons to speak for themselves concerning their social predicament, rather than harnessing their lives to the research machinery of others? This question, we believe, must be asked of even the most "radicalized" and "politicized" research regimens. In this way it becomes possible to make sense of some of the wholly new discourses that have arisen in largely wealthy, Western, industrialized countries over the past few decades.

There are signs in our own historical moment that some eugenic- or countereugenic-inspired formulas of disability are weakening, particularly the rise of new disability art, video, and activism that has fueled revolutionary ways of thinking about disability. The British philosopher John Berger argues that the much-painted figure of nude Vanity in art history tells us more about the desires of the (usually male) artist than it does about "women's narcissism"; in the same way, we claim that eugenics-based beliefs are an imposition of non-disability-identified researchers on disabled peoples' bodies. Recently, during a preliminary thesis defense of a disability studies student, the disabled poet Jim Ferris asked almost bemusedly: "Are there tangible signs that disability is being loosed from its moorings in pathos, pity, tragedy, and dysfunction?" To which the student responded, "No, not necessarily." This was a moment of honest worry about the efficacy of disability art and disability studies for achieving social change. Yet, in a sense it does not matter whether old ideas about disability are or are not on their way out, because there is still much to be learned from the historical inquiry into the roots of what has been an unsettling century and a half of rabid segregation—and even extermination—of disabled people in much of Europe and the United States. The cultural locations of disability help to begin a phase of historical reconstruction that demonstrates that our current approaches to disability are haunted by phantoms of the past—in terms of both literal intellectual lines of descent and reactions to this heritage.

In writing this book we have had a great deal of assistance and critical encouragement. First we recognize students in the master's and Ph.D. program in disability studies at the University of Illinois at Chicago: Meenu Bhambhani, Mike Gill, Michelle Jarman, Eunjung Kim, Sharon Lamp, Yangling "Millie" Li, Heather Stone, Terri Thrower, Sara Vogt, Pam Wheelock, and others. Each provided helpful ideas in disability topics and a sustaining investment in the value of disability studies analysis for us in and out of graduate seminar. Many performed the behind-the-scenes physical labor upon which this book is ultimately based and we thank them for that contribution. Further, we acknowledge the courage of these individuals during trying times when the program was under assault from various quarters of the non–disability studies universe. Their commitment to bettering the program and the university as a safe space for disabled students after them was truly remarkable.

Mark Sherry, Sander Gilman, Ron Amundson, Nirmala Erevelles, Brenda Brueggemann, Tobin Siebers, Michael Davidson, Sarah Rose, and several anonymous readers provided a host of commentary on the manuscript or on the ideas we were developing in tandem with their own original thinking in the field. The Chicago Artists' Coalition—Susan Nussbaum, Riva Lehrer, Jude Martin, Mike Ervin, Tekki Lomnicki, Alana Wallace, and Ginger Lane—as well as Kristi Kirschner and colleagues at the Center for the Study of Disability Ethics, provided a rigorous forum for intellectual debate and creative vision about disability during the development of this book. Literature, art, film, narrative, the sea—all therapy *sometimes*: "whenever it is a damp, drizzly November in my soul . . . whenever my hypos get such an upper hand of me, that it requires a strong moral principle to prevent me from deliberately stepping into the street, and methodically knocking people's hats off—then, I account it high time to get to sea as soon as I can."

In addition, we acknowledge our disability studies cohorts—Michael Berube, Jim Charlton, Eli Clare, Lennard Davis, Jim Ferris, Devva Kasnitz, Georgina Kleege, Simi Linton, Alex Lubet, Robert McRuer, Helen Meekosha, M. Miles, Mike Oliver, Suzanne Poirier, Mark Priestley, Carrie Sandahl, Tom Shakespeare, Margrit Shildrick, Sandy Sufian, James Trent, Sarah Triano, Anne Waldschmidt, Linda Ware, Brian Zimmerman, and many others. Without their willingness to challenge our thinking this book would be even more flawed. We thank each of them for the years of thought they have devoted to the transformation of disability within and outside of the confines of cultural locations identified herein. Without them this line of inquiry would not have been possible.

Additionally, we would like to thank the DAAD "T4 and the Legacies of Eugenics" seminar associates for making a month in Germany seem like the crafting of a utopian space in the midst of a devastating history. It was an amazing experience and the gathering came at a time when we most needed to resolidify our own disability commitments. Potsdam will never be the same thanks to Adrienne Asch, Brenda Brueggemann, Sally Chivers, Sumi Colligan, Nancy Hansen, Ingrid Hofmann, Kanta Kochlar-Lindgren, Nicole Markotic, Emma Mitchell, Debjani Mukherjee, Gerald O'Brien, Sandy O'Neill, Walton Schalick, Mark Sherry, Rosemarie Garland Thomson, Sara Vogt, and Pam Wheelock. Also, thanks to many who took time out of their busy schedules to meet with us during the visit, including Petra Fuchs, Uta George, Katrin Grubar, Uta Hoffman, Swantje Koebsell, Volker van der Locht, Rebecca Maskos, Frank Sobich, Michael Swartze, Mortiz Toffler (and, virtually, Hannelore Witkofski), and Anne Waldschmidt. Their hospitality and commitment to exploring the history of disability in Germany galvanized our own interests ever further!

Douglas Mitchell, executive editor at the University of Chicago Press, fortuitously has sought out intersections across minority inhabitation of urban spaces and sectors. He has been thoughtful and generous in all respects. Timothy McGovern communicates swiftly and followed up on each detail. One never knows whether to apologize to a copy editor or invoke the plausibility of karma.

Some of the material in this book appeared previously in the journals *Disability and Society* and *Patterns of Prejudice*. The idea for a chapter on disability sensations in film was first generated for a report that Barbara Duncan compiled as a result of the first international disability film festival in Moscow in 2002. We are grateful for the role she has played, however marked by global distance, in finding forums for our labor, as well as to others in disability film communities. Cheryl Marie Wade in her support of Superfest, and Denise Roza and Bruce Curtis with Perspectiva, deserve special mention, as do countless others in this burgeoning disability culture undertaking. Lively audiences at the summer seminar on the cultural study of disability in 2003 at the University of Costa Rica focused on the necessity of critiquing disability exclusions across borders. Thanks to Roxana Stupp for paving the way for this vital interchange. Audiences at the Society for Disability Studies, as always, provide the best dissent, dialogue, and momentum. We are forever grateful to live, breathe, work, and reside in proximity to everyone at Chicago's Access Living, Progress Center for Independent Living, and Not Dead Yet.

Finally, we extend our love to our two wonderful children—Cameron and Emma. Without them this work would be meaningless.

CULTURAL

LOCATIONS OF

DISABILITY

Cultural Locations of Disability

DEFINING DISABILITY LOCALES This book examines cultural spaces that have been set out exclusively on behalf of disabled citizens, such as nineteenth-century charity systems; institutions for the feebleminded during the eugenics period; the international disability research industry; sheltered work-shops for the "multi-handicapped"; medically based and documentary film representations of disability; and current academic research trends on disability. We characterize these sites as *cultural locations of disability* in which disabled people find themselves deposited, often against their will.[1] At the very least, each of these locales represents a saturation point of content about disability that has been produced by those who share certain beliefs about disability as an aspect of human differences. We trace these beliefs back to the eugenics era, when disability began to be construed as an undesirable deviation from normative existence. Even in the face of benign rhetoric about disabled people's best interests, these locations of disability have resulted in treatment, both in the medical and cultural sense, that has proven detrimental to their meaningful participation in the invention of culture itself. The chapters that follow demonstrate how *these locations exist largely at odds with the collective and individual well-being of disabled people.*[2]

To demonstrate this undermining of collective well-being, we distinguish the locations under study here from more authenticating cultural modes of disability knowledge, such as the disability rights movement, disability culture, the independent living movement, and other experientially based organizations of disabled people.[3] These sites are critical to the growing social recognition and analysis of disabled people's situation in the United States and elsewhere. In fact, a critique of these eugenic locations comes into being largely in the wake of the development of politicized disability efforts. Without these politicized efforts to reclaim disability as something more than tragedy, dysfunction, and misfortune, we would not be able to fully comprehend the entrapment of these other cultural locations.[4] Thus, this book finds its basis in the understandings made available by disability activist and cultural studies models. These arenas of politicized endeavor occupy an alternative ground without which these critiques could not be articulated.[5] Our analyses here seek not to fill in an alternative "positive" content of disability experience, for that would merely replace one form of historical simplification with another, but rather to destabilize our dominant ways of knowing disability. Alternative ways of comprehending disabled bodies and minds are often best explained within experiential forms, such as personal narratives, performance art, and films, rather than in the often objectifying realms of "research" about disabled people. We explicitly lay out this argument in our concluding chapters on Fred Wiseman's disability documentary cinema and the institutionalization of disability studies in the U.S. academy.

One of our primary tasks in the chapters that follow is to demonstrate how these institutional, and largely scientific, ways of knowing disability can be challenged from a historical perspective. Second, in recreating some significant aspects of disability history, we seek to undermine the presumption that U.S. culture has produced an "objective" discourse about disabled bodies. Rather than *locations*, then, this book could refer to *dis-locations*; particularly if we take the latter term to mean the degree to which disability results in a person's active disenfranchisement from levels of participation and experience afforded to most other citizens. Each of the institutions under analysis in this book forms a link in the chain of complicity that colludes (knowingly or unknowingly) to limit the freedoms and mobility of people with disabilities. These locations of disability form the foundation of a quintessentially modernist project. Their *modus operandi* consists of efforts to classify and pathologize human differences (known today as disabilities) and then manage them through various institutional locations. While often parading under the humanist guise of help or sympathy for "the unfortunate," they accomplish their debilitating effects through taxonomies of naming, the statistical calculation of average and nonstandard bodies, restrictive public policy implementation, and especially participation in a normative science of eugenic origin. The eugenics period provided the tools and rationale for a hygienic drive toward the valorization of perfection and normalization.[6] These goals stand at the heart of the modernist impulse.[7] Rather than make eugenics an aberration of modernism, this study takes as the targets of our critique the practices of hereditary "cleansing" developed in this period.

By refiguring eugenics in this manner, our book delves into a little explored history of people with disabilities in the United States—or rather, engages in what Longmore and Umansky refer to as the need in disability studies to fill in profound "historiological gaps" (2001, 3). Beginning in the mid-nineteenth century and ending with present-day research and representational practices, this study identifies key institutions and networks that have helped to define American attitudes toward human bodies: not merely disabled bodies and their nearly exclusive association with stigma and dysfunction, but rather *all* bodies in the sense that disability is viewed as excessive hardship in the manifestation of human variation. Or, to shift disciplinary models for a moment, we may note that in a scientific bell curve scenario, disabled bodies are most often located at the extreme tails of statistical measures of deviation (Canguilhem 1991, 265; Hacking 1990, 169).

As a result, the devaluation of disabled bodies places in jeopardy all bodies that exist within proximity to "deviance" (and ultimately no body escapes this relation), particularly given that in modernity the cultivation of technologies geared to identify deviance begins to inform the very conceptualization of embodiment. To salvage the danger that deviance poses generally, designations of disability seek to place some populations as not only anomalous to, but nearly outside of, cultural adjudications of functional, aesthetic, and biological value.[8] Additionally, the operation of deviance identified here helps to explain why those who associate in nonhierarchical ways with disabled people also threaten wider cultural efforts to cordon off disability from the continuum of human embodiment.

DISABILITY AS A CULTURAL MODEL As a consequence of this cultural positioning of disability at the extremes of social value, we utilize in this book what has come to be called a "cultural model" of disability: one primarily associated with social science–based and humanities-based disability studies discourses in the United States (Longmore and Goldberger 2000; Jarman et al. 2002). To stake a claim to the particulars of disability studies epistemologies at work in the cultural model, we approach our task by comparing our own methods with those of the social model developed largely in the United Kingdom, beginning with the history of the Union of Physically Impaired Against Segregation (UPIAS).[9] The British discourse on disability both preceded and substantively influenced U.S. models. In part, our efforts here seek to respond to continuing claims (mostly accurate) that disability studies in the United States has yet to articulate its own analytical methods distinct from those of the British social model practitioners (Barnes 1999, 577). Although we cannot perform this task in an exhaustive way, since, as in Britain, there are numerous versions of disability studies practices within the cultural model, we can offer some observations about our own understanding of shared methodological assumptions. In doing so we make a foray into the necessary articulation of founding beliefs that underwrite alternative disability studies methods with respect to the dominant paradigms in the field (for example, social model analyses). The goal here is not to codify these practices as monolithic—a project that would inevitably and rightly fail—but rather to begin addressing the question directly since we do believe that there are common tenets in cultural model scholarship that designate a coherent array of approaches.

The best way to define an alternative model is to identify how it differs from other predecessor models—in this case, the "social model of disability." The trend in disability studies for years has been to distinguish between disability and impairment, arguing that the latter term is a neutral designator of biological difference while the former represents a social process termed "disablement" (Oliver 1983, 23; Crow 1996, 206–7; Morris 2001, 4). This study follows a different theoretical framework. "Disability" in this book—in keeping with current formulations informed by cultural and identity studies—is largely, but not strictly synonymous with sites of cultural oppression. It does not solely represent the social coordinates, as Liz Crow puts it, of restraints "that we must escape" (1996, 206). Instead, our use of this term is much closer to that offered by scholars such as Sally French (1994), Simi Linton (1998), and others who recognize disability as a site of phenomenological value that is not purely synonymous with the processes of social disablement. Such an emphasis does not hide the degree to which social obstacles and biological capacities may impinge upon our lives, but rather suggests that the result of those differences comes to bear significantly on the ways disabled people experience their environments and their bodies. Environment and bodily varia-

6

tion (particularly those traits experienced as socially stigmatized differences) inevitably impinge upon each other. Thus, as the Canadian philosopher Susan Wendell points out, "the distinction between the biological reality of disability and the social construction of a disability cannot be made sharply" (1996, 35). The definition of disability must incorporate both the outer and inner reaches of culture and experience as a combination of profoundly social and biological forces.

Some of the key theorists in disability studies have overlooked opportunities to theorize this interactional space between embodiment and social ideology. Strict social model adherents often refer to the biological and cognitive manifestations of difference as "impairment" in order to situate the phenomenon outside of the concerns of disability studies. Similarly, the therapies have also sought to retain the use of the term "impairment" because it allows an interactional space to exist between bodies and society while continuing to allow disability to be referenced as dysfunction in need of intervention. One can witness this contemporary approach to impairment in the machinations of the WHO's disability assessment scale, where environment is taken into account but individual impairments continue to result in demerits for an overall quality of life rating. Goffman's (1986) theory of stigma and Butler's (1999) deconstruction of sex/gender binaries have been influential to cultural model discourses because they formulate theories of passing, psychic formation, and materiality as social processes. Cultural model approaches likewise tend to recognize identity and body as constructed. Such distinctions are still naturalized in fields such as psychology and psychiatry as organic to those who exist within imperiled bodies. In this way we can begin to understand the theoretical move to identity politics that early cultural approaches in disability studies took up.

These emphases in a "cultural model of disability" prove important because we do not, for instance, assume an absent relationship between therapeutic beliefs about disability and disabled people's experience. The two inform each other, for better or worse, and consequently we must begin to theorize the degree to which a dominant discourse such as rehabilitation science comes to be internalized by disabled people. This relationship first took shape during the eugenics period in institutions for the "feebleminded." Bodies still subject to normalization schemes find themselves disciplined with respect to the performance of skills and functions that are alien to them (or outside of their grasp): people with mobility impairments are videotaped for a visual record of an abnormal gait (one that is later viewed by physical therapists and orthopedists in the absence of the individual about whom the record is made); variations in small motor skills that attend cerebral palsy result in endless rounds of fitting beads onto a string; those with head injuries are subject to memorization tasks; hearing-impaired individuals are given batteries of audiological exams; and, most of all, a few evaluations are never enough. One finds oneself endlessly subject to a seemingly inexhaustible evaluation regimen.

Rehabilitation often *subjects* limitations in functional capacities to the very activities that exist outside of a body's abilities. This emphasis on "inability" is the result of a persistent historical attention to formulations of disability as excessive functional deficit. Such an approach results in the development of programs of repetitious self-care in which the ritualistic preparation of the body becomes the largest horizon of training for disabled people. What is the psychic toll of repetitiously attempting to perform activities beyond one's ability? These tasks are largely assigned from the "acute" period of disability, when rehabilitation patients are most likely to feel nostalgia for a return to prior functionality; in the case of congenital disabilities, the rehabilitation disciplines target children stripped of personal autonomy to make their own rehabilitation choices.

This is one reason why merely consulting with disabled people about their own desires is not a remedy to a history of diminished autonomy (Barnes 2003, 5). Recent trends to consult disabled people on their own desires, such as "emancipatory research" and "client-centered care," do not evade the social problematic at the heart of disability: if disabled people are subject to the internalization of dominant definitions and values of disability just like those who are nondisabled, then asking clients about their personal goals is not a pat solution to more humane models of intervention. This is particularly relevant given that rehabilitation stubbornly clings to the "acute medical phase" as a baseline for designating what "disabled people want," as if there was a universal possibility of filling in the blank for such a diverse population. Such an approach belies the necessity of interrogating therapeutic inattention to the internalization of dominant ideologies about disability. The rehabilitation regimen becomes little more than a return to the site of the wound that disability has become; one of the few means for paying attention to disability is individual behavior associated with this wounding process as the source of one's psychic organization. Ignoring this domain effectively allows rehabilitation providers and researchers to justify their own practices without acknowledging that they capitalize on a transitional phase of impairment inevitably subject to change. What would happen if rehabilitation decided to base its intervention strategies on long-term goals of value to people living with disabilities, developed after the primary period of adjustment? How would our rehabilitation industry work if it were not based so exclusively on elusive principles of normalcy (or prior levels of functionality) that, by definition of one's impairment, cannot be regained?

Recent attempts to include a social context as a factor in "impaired functionality measures" do little to ameliorate the normalization dilemma. As has been carefully documented in disability studies literature, the original International Classification of Impairments, Disabilities and Handicaps (ICIDH) was roundly rejected by disability groups on the basis of its grounding in the medicalization of disability as individual pathology (Oliver 1990; Coleridge 1993; Pfeiffer 2000). The new ICIDH 2 aims to improve upon the solely functional emphasis of the International Classification of Functioning (ICF) and ICIDH 1 by adding a social component to each of its three main categories of assessment: impairment (body function and structure); activity (that which used to be disability); and participation. Because the assessment tool factors environmental influences into its degree of impairment calculation, the ICIDH 2 has been proclaimed a "universal" paradigm by its authors. Within this revised model disability still retains its status as a *health* concern as opposed to a political situation, and therefore, its remediation continues to be imagined as interventions performed upon normative bodies and their environments. Besides failing to attend to the myriad differences across cultures, identities, and time periods, the ICIDH 2 may ultimately only further depoliticize disability due to its generation of "objective," numerical measures about bodies. These are all efforts of a research industry trying to retain the necessity of functional measures set to various regionally specific tasks (based largely on overdeveloped world criteria) without regard to geographical or cultural particularity. In this book we seek to examine the ways in which the cultural locations of disability dramatically affect the formulation of bodily, sensory, and cognitive differences in social and scientific realms. Our aim is to show how institutions that control people with disabilities are mediated through a manipulation of material, social, and environmental contexts.

In contrast to the ICIDH 2, the application of a "cultural model" recognizes one aspect of disability as a politicized self-naming strategy that distances people with disabilities from dominant definitions of incapacity and dysfunction. The term *disability* recognizes that there exists a necessary distance between dominant cultural perspectives of disability (sometimes signified as "handicap") as tragic embodiment and a politically informed disability-subculture perspective that seeks to define itself against devaluing mainstream views of disability. In this sense, the cultural model of disability acknowledges a split in the term *impairment* while the social model tends to cast off "impairment" as neutral bodily difference (Finkelstein 1996; Barnes 1996). Rather than lacking a term exclusively referring to "social disadvantage," the cultural model has an understanding that impairment is both human variation encountering environmental obstacles *and* socially mediated difference that lends group identity and phenomenological perspective. The significance of this formulation can be understood through stories about disability such as *Oedipus Rex*, where the limping Oedipus solves the sphinx's riddle *because* of his experience with mobility impairment (Mitchell and Snyder 2000, 61). This insight shifts disability from either a medical pathology or signifier of social discrimination into a source of embodied revelation. Such a recognition permits a more complex understanding of disability experience, without the ready depth or easy sentimentality offered by charity and popular film. In recognizing this split in the conceptualization of impairment, the cultural model of disability does not jettison embodiment but views it as a potentially meaningful materiality. An embodied experience can be embraced while also resulting in social discrimination and material effects (such as pain, discomfort, or incapacity).

In cultural model applications, this divided understanding of impairment is encompassed by the larger, politicized term *disability*. The dual operation of the term is why many cultural model scholars understand "disability" to function both as a referent for a process of social exposé and as a productive locus for identification. Thus, disability is once removed from impairment in that the concept depends upon both conditions of impairment being met—namely embodied difference (this also may be due to a "socially perceived" phenomenon as designated in the Americans with Disabilities Act) that precipitates social discrimination (since not all impairments result in social disenfranchisement, due to mitigating factors such as class, insufficient "monstrosity," and so forth). We believe the cultural model provides a fuller concept than the social model, in which "disability" signifies only discriminatory encounters. The formulation of a cultural model allows us to theorize a political act of renaming that designates disability as a site of resistance and a source of cultural agency previously suppressed—at least to the extent that groups can successfully rewrite their own definition in view of a damaging material and linguistic heritage. The sites of this suppression and the processes by which they are implemented are the subject of this book.

A significant part of renaming as a form of resistance involves the interrogation of medical labels themselves as fuzzy, historical, and often stigmatizing artifacts of biology and cognition as social constructs. The social model of disability articulated in Britain by UPIAS (1976), Mike Oliver (1983), and others, for instance, seeks to undermine the legitimacy of medical and rehabilitation discourses about disabled bodies by ruling them out of bounds: "disability is wholly and exclusively social . . . disability [has] nothing to do with the body. It is a consequence of social oppression" (quoted in Schriempf 2001, 59). Likewise, as Shelley Tremain argues, by ignoring impairment the social model leaves intact the power/knowledge nexus that defines and interprets impairment (2002, 33–34). Such an approach situates these domains as relatively untouched and undertheorized sources of disability oppression (Shakespeare and Watson 1995; Hughes and Paterson 1997; Corker 1999). Rather than cordon off medicine and therapy as arenas of the body tangential to disability studies concerns, this book takes up discourses of the body that developed within normalization systems as locations in need of specific sociohistorical analysis.

BIOLOGICAL AND SOCIAL WORTH While some disability studies scholars have criticized the "social model" for failing to address the reality of biological, cognitive, and sensory deficiencies, many disability writers and cultural studies theorists have challenged the very empiricism informing medical conditions and labels. For instance, Ian Hacking (2000) has argued that while science may eventually locate an organic cause for a condition such as autism (although he seems highly skeptical of such claims), this would do little to counter the more powerful social contexts that we have now created around those diagnosed with autism. In this scenario, for instance, special education classrooms have so internalized the standard, one-size-fits-all medical definition of autism that the educational context itself produces "acting out" behaviors with a fair amount of consistency (Hacking 2000, 110). For Hacking, a "feedback loop" develops, in which the medical label of autism begins to interact with those assigned the diagnosis. Consequently, people with autism may resist or internalize the designation (or, perhaps more usually, some combination of these two options). The label itself presupposes a "type" of population that then prompts efforts to refashion identities in response to the initial diagnostic parameters. In a more banal example of looping, disability scholars and activists frequently encounter journalists who seem to believe that gaining access to one's disability label somehow delivers the truth of one's social identity (and thus one's political motivations). Instead, participants in these groups often find themselves resisting the effort to identify their diagnoses, in order to complicate medical definitions with the more nuanced stories of their own experience (Rubin

2000; Mairs 1998; Clare 1999; Michalko 2002). This tactic of drawing from one's own experience shows once again how a cultural model of disability provides an opportunity to reimagine the landscape of impairment as well as its attendant social contexts.

Given the powerful influence in the United States of civil rights movements organized around feminist, racial, and queer identities, disability studies has inevitably adopted many of the strategies and tactics of these political movements. Key concepts and methods of those discourses have come into disability studies as a way of extending the analytical terrain for discussing disability as a social issue. Readers will find in this work and others the implementation of such concepts as passing, binary systems, biologism, representation, naturalization, segregation, patriarchy, racism, and so forth. Each of these theoretical issues comes replete with its own methodological and philosophical innovations to which one can also apply disability. Rather than add disability to the theoretical matrices of other marginalized peoples, we argue in this book that disability has become the keystone in the edifice of bodily based inferiority rationales built up since the late eighteenth century. For it was at this historical moment in Europe and the United States that, as Michel Foucault observes, "a technology of human abnormality, a technology of abnormal individuals appears precisely when a regular network of knowledge and power has been established" (2003, 61). Abnormality has a history, and by designating a specific historical moment of arrival, Foucault demonstrates that the appearance of pathological bodies is dependent upon techniques of identification (classification systems of normalcy and deviance). Within the cultural model disability functions not as an identification of abnormality but rather as a tool of cultural diagnosis. It provides a way of understanding how formulas of abnormality develop and serve to discount entire populations as *biologically inferior.*

To take just three quick historical examples of disability as the foundation of biological ideologies of inferiority, think of Charles Darwin's use of racial primitives and cognitively disabled people as evolutionary throwbacks of "man"; early feminist efforts to draw equivalences between women's "weaker" bodies and those of people with physical disability; and Karl Marx's use of crippling capitalism as a producer of the emasculated bodies of disabled laborers. The three key examples from history identified here provide further contextualization of the use of disability by various nineteenth-century liberation movements: Darwin in his works on evolution uses an equation between "primitive" racial cultures and people with cognitive disability as an anchor for his argument about evolving human traits. Since

Nordic Caucasians occupy a pinnacle of development in the evolution of human species from animals, race and disability serve as ways by which Darwin references evidence for the existence of "earlier" states of man. Darwin's use of races and disabled people as evolutionary throwbacks (or static evolutionary examples) establishes them as akin to a human fossil bed. Their manifestation of "regressive" traits signifies a prior moment in the evolutionary progress of humankind that still bears the traces of a less sophisticated developmental past. While other evolutionary systems, such as that devised by Galton and later eugenicists, referenced disability as a deviance existing along the bell curve of mental and physiological capacities shared by any given population, Darwin relies on what he believes to be the "rudimentary forms" of these types of human animals on his hierarchical scale. This is in spite of his earlier argument, in *On the Origin of Species*, against a progressive fantasy of history and in favor of variations as for "the good of the species." Between the publication of *Origin* in 1859 and *Descent of Man* in 1871, Darwin's theories moved toward support of the growing eugenics movement that would equate racialized and disabled bodies with undesirable biological deviances.

Likewise, early feminist reformers, such as Victoria Woodhull and Tennie Claflin, referenced the bodies of disabled men as a justification against women as the weaker sex. In their 1871 *Woodhull and Claflin's Weekly*, they discount physiological strength as an appropriate barometer for denial of the vote to women because such an assumption would effectively strip certain men of their rights within an electoral system: "[The weaker physique of the average woman] is a curious reason for the subordination of the woman; since in a just application it would defeat itself, in depriving every physically feeble or ailing or crippled man—no matter what his moral or intellectual status—of the vote, and placing the same in the hand of every amazon, virago, termagant—no matter how coarse or ignorant—if they could but muscularly grasp it" (*Woodhull and Claflin's Weekly* 1871). While the Darwinian argument hinged upon the idea of populations as biological throwbacks, Woodhull and Claflin's analysis uses disability to argue that physical capacity should be no basis for policy formation. At the same time that it seemed to accept the patriarchal determinism embodied in the idea of women as the weaker sex, second-wave feminism argued that if male disability (presumably an indicator of "weaker" physiologies) was not viewed as a disqualifier, neither should gender be so viewed. This argument, of course, avoided the fact that institutionalized disabled people were debarred from voting as well, due to their segregated cultural location.

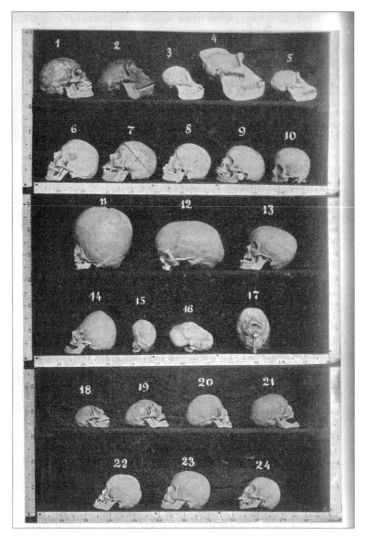

CABINET OF COMPARATIVE SKULL "DEFORMITIES" FROM RACIAL "PRIMITIVES"
AND DISABLED PEOPLE

On another track, the noted writer Charlotte Perkins Gilman—who was also an avowed eugenicist, along with other leading feminists, such as Margaret Sanger and Josephine Donovan—used disability as synonymous with corruption. Borrowing from the well-worn nineteenth-century trope of the female invalid, Gilman argued that incarceration in the domestic sphere led to the production of inferior children: "The female segregated to the uses of sex alone naturally deteriorates in racial development, and naturally transmits that deterioration to her offspring. The human mother, in the processes of reproduction, shows no gain in efficiency over the lower animals, but rather a loss, and so far presents no evidence to prove that her specialization to sex is of any advantage to her young. The mother of a dead baby or the baby of a dead mother; the sick baby, the crooked baby, the idiot baby; the exhausted, nervous, prematurely aged mother,—these are not uncommon among us; and they do not show much progress in our motherhood" (1998 [1898], 90–91).

By using the extremist vocabulary of eugenics to forward disability as a threat against the violence of patriarchal restrictions, Gilman effectively identified the scourge of disability as a product of female immobility and insufficient educational opportunity. In addition, the argument also cites evolutionary arguments based on pangenesis, according to which it was possible to pass on regressive traits that were acquired or purely social in nature. Limits on women's participation in the male world manifested themselves in the production of "inferior" progeny who then, in turn, diminished the nation's hereditary stock.

While early feminist arguments invoked the social privileges of handicapped men as a rationale for women's rights or used eugenic rhetoric as a threat, class analyses hinged on an equation between disability and capitalist corruption. For Marx (1906), the "crippling of the working class body" by capitalist greed became pivotal to his analysis. Rather than cite disability as a form of human deviance, he deployed bodily incapacity, disease, and debilitation as his primary evidence for the usurpation of physical labor by capital: "Some crippling of body and mind is inseparable even from division of labour in society as a whole. Since, however, manufacture carries this social separation of branches of labour much further, and also, by its peculiar division, attacks the individual at the very roots of his life, it is the first to afford the materials for, and to give a start to, industrial pathology" (50). If capitalism and cripples were sometimes inexorably linked (as we argue in our first chapter), class analyses depended on an equation of labor capacity with the national citizen. In eugenics, arguments about the ability to labor were also used, but only by way of invalidating people with disabilities on the basis of their failed labor skills. The Marxist or class-based argument bemoaned disability as a stripping of capacity from the body by excessive labor demands; rising levels of worker disability thus provided a reliable indicator of the corruption of capital.

For instance, Marx relies heavily on government reports of unhealthy working conditions to shore up the brutality of a profit-based system: "The sanitary officers, the industrial inquiry commissioners, the factory inspectors, all . . . declare that consumption and other lung diseases among the workpeople are necessary conditions to the existence of capital" (1906, 215). Much like arguments in favor of Darwinian evolution in the nineteenth century, analyses of capitalism moved the production of disability to the front and center of their proofs. Marx's analyses, consequently, denounced the creation of disability while solidifying the concept of labor capacity as the foundation of citizenship rights. As we argue in chapter 2, this presumption of the ability to labor as a cornerstone of human validity would serve as a key impetus for the segregation of disabled people throughout this period. In each of these examples, one recognizes the growing utility of disability to various liberation ideologies cultivated in the nineteenth century.

In making this argument about the foundational role of disability in oppressive biological schemes, we seek to show that disability studies has benefited by adopting the theoretical strategies of other minority discourses while also enduring the stigma of its association with the "reality" of human dysfunctionality within those traditions. One of the major arguments of this book is that disability has been historically fashioned as if it were a denotative designation of biologically based deficits. "Biological worth" has been continually conflated with "social worth" as if one's own body referenced the extent to which one could meaningfully participate in and contribute to culture-making (Desrosiers 2002, 114–15).

One of the best and most devastating examples of this tendency to equate biological and social worth occurs in Sir Francis Galton's work on hereditary genius (1869). By associating a masculinist model of intellectual accomplishment with familial hereditary patterns, Galton made a key linkage between biological determinism and the significance of an individual's social contribution. This proved the critical step in the fashioning of eugenics ideology toward disabled, ethnic, and sexual Others. Galton attempted to argue that the purpose of his study was "to make manifest the great and measurable differences between mental and bodily functions of individuals, and to prove that the laws of heredity are as applicable to the former as to the latter" (2001 [1869], 35). Thus, intellectual capacities, like physical capacities, proved inheritable, and an individual's social value was deterministically guaranteed from birth. Within this model of hereditary genius, people with cognitive and physical disabilities (particularly those labeled as "idiots" in the early nineteenth century and "feebleminded" in the late nineteenth century) failed socially as a result of their inferior hereditary stock. Galton describes it as "those who are the least efficient in physical, intellectual, and moral grounds, forming our lowest class, and those who are the most efficient forming our highest class" (2001 [1869], 37). Disability, gender, ethnic, and/or racial affiliation did not preclude social achievement, but rather functioned as a reliable predictive marker for those who could not transcend their biological limitations within a stratified class-based system.[10]

We intend to follow disability studies and other minority discourses in the absolute refutation of this parallel between biological and social worth. The infusion of civil rights and identity-based movements into disability studies has helped develop theoretical sophistication and has allowed these terms to take on their own distinctiveness within discourses of disability. For instance, references of passing to questions of color hierarchies and performances of heterosexuality within queer contexts are further transformed within a disability context as sites of resistance to cultural demands for normalization (Stiker 1999, 135; McRuer 2003, 87; Sandahl 2003). Yet there is also significant conflict in these cross-cultural and disciplinary comparisons. Race, feminist, and queer studies have all participated to one degree or another in a philosophical lineage that seeks to distance those social categories from more "real" biological incapacities (Mitchell and Snyder 1997, 6).[11] Thus, in order to counteract charges of deviance historically assigned to blackness, femininity, or homosexuality, these political discourses have tended to reify disability as "true" insufficiency, thereby extricating their own populations from equations of inferiority. This mode is most recently evidenced in a book by Nancy Ordover (2003) titled *American Eugenics: Race, Queer Anatomy, and the Science of Nationalism.* Although the author includes disability as one disenfranchised community among others in this period, her chapters focus exclusively on questions of race, gender, and sexuality as the maligned identities of the eugenics movement. The exploration of *identity crossings* between disability, race, class, gender, and queer identities forms a significant part of the contribution that cultural model disability scholars can make to the field. As a part of this tradition of inquiry, we take up the intersections of some of these culturally imposed conditions in the following chapters.

We reexamine disability experiences in the United States and Europe from an analysis of the history of normalization schemes. This entails scrutiny of a continuum of bodies and body-based beliefs in the medical, rehabilitation, aesthetic, and cultural registers. In each of the historical examples mentioned above, the inherent definition of disability as bodily based incapacity underwrites various civil rights agendas. From the late eighteenth century onward, the disabled body was increasingly situated as a common denominator of disenfranchisement. This general observation about an entrenched political rhetoric of disability serves as a useful example of the fraught terrain occupied by formal ableism. We associate ableism with ideological formulas that equate devalued bodily conditions with decreased social value. This book might be described as an effort to understand how a concept, such as disability exclusively formulated as human liability, remains fundamental to arguments about "in-built inferiority": a purportedly biological feature that mires a group of individuals in a devalued condition that cannot be overcome, trained away, or transcended to any significant degree (Fredrickson 2002, 5). During a recent conference on the dual status of race and disability, held in Utah, people of color and disabled people compared notes on their experiences and recognized "much common ground," including "poverty, discrimination, lack of political clout, and, sometimes, a public backlash created by perceptions that [both groups] get special treatment" (Griggs 2003). This intertwined heritage of social disapprobation occurs because contemporary U.S. culture has imbibed a heady brew of eugenic beliefs in biology as destiny.

BIOLOGICAL OUTCASTS Chapter 1 explains the practice of group differentiation as a matter of partitioning the deserving from the undeserving poor. The "undeserving" are those who do not try hard enough. This historical practice has repercussions in contemporary global urban centers of making disabled bodies the deficient ones that merit donations for the sake of their bodily suffering (Stone 1984, 21). This practice extends from the badging laws of charitable giving to the apparent benefit of "qualifying" for a handicap parking pass. We discuss these historically generated and highly "natural" means for serving disabled persons as a way to think about strategies employed for the control and management of disability that have been exported and enforced across human societies to one degree or another.[12] Throughout this book, we view labels as a matter of discursive production and policy rationale rather than of empirical accuracy, as names of convenience and attitudinal repositories more than as sites of reclamation created from what the disabled performance artist Cheryl Marie Wade calls "the inside-out" (*Vital Signs* [film] 1995).

Examples of the detrimental labeling phenomenon given in this book provide a glimpse into historical attitudes toward disability and thus function as lessons in how scientific and medical categories come replete with stigmatizing beliefs. These terms of identification include "cripples," "evolutionary throwbacks," "feebleminded," "cretins," "idiots," "criminals," "delinquents," and "defectives." Such terms gave way to more contemporary acronyms of "multi-handicap" such as MR (mental retardation), CP (cerebral palsy), MD (muscular dystrophy), DD (developmental disability), and a bevy of other dislocated letters from the alphabet, now nearly shorn of their references to material biologies. If a system needs an abbreviation to refer to its object of study, then there is something wrong with the root word itself.[13]

In the eugenics era, and still today, groups of bodies that house disabilities sport labels that epitomize the idea that disability marks people off as exceptionally, even dramatically, unsuitable in comparison to those occupying the bulky middle of the bell curve—the domain of normalcy constituted by quantitative measures of human appearances and capacities. Terms such as "feebleminded," "subnormal," "noneducable," "crippled," "defective," "monstrous," and "unfit" once infused popular media and served as professional diagnoses. Yet one era's "scientific" designations become another era's derogatory epithets. The updated eugenics of the present day, often called genetics, examines conditions in bodies that are classed as "mutant," "tragic," "coding errors," "suffering," "unhealthy," "deviant," "faulty," and "abnormal." Our measurement instruments continue to seek to monitor and predict the fate of disabled persons presumably tagging along at the tail end of statistical deviation curves. But in each of the terms one finds an already assigned subjective judgment about the value of human variation. In this sense the terms cannot function as empirical accounts of difference and adaptation. They arrive complete with a denigrating sentiment undergirding cultural responses to disability. Biology is destiny when the rhetoric leaps from a descriptive register to a presumption of undesirability in need of erasure. The particular kind of social erasure we analyze in this book is that where disabled citizens are forced to exchange their liberty for necessary (and unnecessary) social supports. Their social removal is predicated upon their receipt of an "assistance" that is calculated to alleviate their misfortune.

That the history presented in the following chapters is almost exclusively detrimental to bodies labeled as disabled is not accidental. We aim to reconstruct crucial moments in the history of U.S. attitudes toward people with disabilities, and in doing so, we examine key locations of disability, such as charity networks, institutions, scientific discourses, sheltered workshops, popular films, and research universities that produce influential social beliefs about disability. We primarily come to know disabled people, both historically and in our own moment, through representations of their lives, experiences, and bodies that have been manufactured by those outside of the immediate disability experience. Unless one seeks out specific gatherings of people with disabilities, operates in allegiance with an independent living center, or is incarcerated along with dozens of one's fellow disabled citizens, one receives cultural perspectives on disability filtered through documents and images at best secondhand to these experiences.

A substantive body of research that tackles the social history of disability in the United States from the point of view of those who embodied the category and, subsequently, lived the experience is still lacking. Thus, we believe that there is much to gain from undertaking an initial review of a voluminous discursive tradition on disability from those who primarily position themselves, out of professional advantage and scientific demand, outside of disability subjectivities.

We think of our efforts in this book as somewhat akin to the drama Virginia Woolf narrates in her investigations of gender inequity in *A Room of One's Own* (1928). Woolf's narrator goes to the university library to research what has been written and thought about women's social status. Much to her surprise, she finds that volumes have been composed on the subject. As a result, her study must be modified so as to explain the abundance of belief, assertion, research, and measurement, all cycling around a curious irony: how can women have exerted such fascination on the "opposite" sex throughout history and yet continue to be identified as the devalued gender? What circumstances lead to cultural devaluation in the midst of an outpouring of textual, statistical, and visual materials on the subject? What does one do when confronted with too many studies and not enough meaningful insight? One is tempted to propose a mathematical formula that the degree of fascination with a cultural object is inversely proportional to the severity of its cultural devaluation. This, at least, is the cultural predicament of disability.

The paradox of devaluation in the midst of perpetual discussion about the meaning and treatment of disability is at the heart of this book. It seeks not just to understand the content of works written about disabled people in the United States during the second industrial era, but also to analyze the reasons that disability has held such fascination—one could even say obsession—among administrators, scientists, government officials, teachers, public health and social workers, psychologists, medical personnel, and rehabilitation workers.

GEOGRAPHIES OF THE UNDESIRABLE In the introduction to our first book, *The Body and Physical Difference*, we argued that unlike many minority groups, disabled people have found themselves marginalized *as a result of* the proliferation of their representation in various discourses (Mitchell and Snyder, eds., 1997, 16–17). This paradox underlies the present work as well. If, for Virginia Woolf, women historically function as a device to reflect the image of men back to themselves at twice their normal size, should we suggest something similar with respect to the cultural function of disability for subjects seeking to establish, by contrast, their abilities? What can we learn about disability by beginning with the premise that our understanding of human variation has been filtered through the perspectives and research of those who locate disability on the outermost margins of human value?

If we now have an established presumption that the object of research cannot adequately assess its conditions objectively because of self-interest and bias, then it seems to us that one can also postulate the inverse — namely, that a tradition of largely detrimental commentary about disability by non-disability-identified researchers results in mountains of research that skews our perspectives on disability in a largely negative way.

Since the advent of the rehabilitation era, disabled people have resided within close proximity to a scientific ethos that misidentifies objectivity with the debasement of its object of study (O'Brien 2001). Consequently, the phenomenon of disability has been routinely represented as the site of undesirability; one that only provides recourse to a battery of interventions involved in the alleviation, diminishment, normalization, oversight, and invasive management of disabled persons' lives. This is not the product of objectivity or sound scientific practice; rather, it is the outgrowth of a history in which disability has functioned as the "obviously" undesirable location in a geography of beliefs that must repeatedly perform their neutrality by reasserting, again and again, this defining undesirability. As the Frankfurt school social theorist Theodor Adorno explains, the repetitive discovery that things were as we thought they were all along is central to today's scientific method: "What is wholly verified empirically, with all the checks demanded by competitors, can always be foreseen by the most modest use of reason. The questions are so ground down in the mill that, in principle, little more can emerge than that the percentage of tuberculosis cases is higher in a slum district than on Park Avenue" (1994, 41). People with disabilities have seen themselves anchor a scientific research industry that continually circles back to some variation on the age-old observation that disability is a misfortune, because our research "reveals" that same point time and time again.

One can now feel safe in saying that disability has become synonymous with many of our most banal cultural recognitions. Today's disability research industry pursues many of the following correlations: disability and unemployment have a high degree of correlation; disabled people rate their own quality of life higher than physicians do; disabled people would rather

live on their own than in institutions; disabled people should be able to exercise because it improves their lifestyle; families often prove detrimental to
people with disabilities; a disabled life is worth living; restricted head movements in infants are a reliable sign of neuromuscular disorder. In theory,
there may be nothing wrong with these studies—except that the research has
been so entrenched in proving disadvantage that imbalance results. Today's
disability science accomplishes this task by trying to prove, as Adorno (1994)
points out, that common-sense observations can be empirically validated.

We therefore adopt a disability studies methodology that exposes the history of subject/object divisions in U.S. disability research. These approaches
unearth the historical imbalance that has informed disability research enterprises. This book queries the impact of ongoing research and service relationships in the United States by examining six key sites of disability scrutiny:
(1) nineteenth-century charity operations; (2) the rise of eugenic science;
(3) international collaboration in restrictive state policies for disabled people during the world wars; (4) the deepening of contemporary segregation
practices for people with "multi-handicaps"; (5) the rise of a new disability
documentary cinema that contests mainstream representational practices;
and (6) the conflicts attendant in recent efforts to institutionalize disability
studies in the American academy. We choose these sites because they unfold
in history as if they were all part of a shared design—one leading to the other
like a fan neatly unfolding one section at a time. They are not the only locations that we might have selected for inclusion here; other researchers have
chosen a variety of alternative locations for similar analyses, such as disabled
veterans policies (Gerber 2000), telethons (Longmore 1997), hospital schools
(Byrom 2001), or disabled pension systems (Stone 1984; *When Billy Broke His
Head* [film] 1995). Our chosen sites specifically involved eugenics beliefs
and practices as either the ostensible or covert informing ideology. They are
not intended to be exhaustive of the locations within which disabled people
find themselves ensconced ("walled off" might be the better term), but they
are intended to represent, when taken collectively, a constellation of restrictive institutional and discursive spaces.

The analysis of these cultural locations allows us to document formative moments in the making of disability into a potent medical and social
classification in the United States. The category is not a given throughout
the country's history; in fact, "disability" as a socially composed grouping is
less than two hundred years old. The relative newness of the rubric helps
to establish our first principle: disability has not automatically engendered
a process of historical singling-out in the United States; rather, to do so is

to participate in a uniquely "modern" preoccupation. As eugenicists such as Henry H. Goddard were fond of pointing out, feeblemindedness (the late nineteenth-century term for disability) is not necessarily feeblemindedness in the country (or in agrarian economic contexts); it comes to the surface when individuals are faced with the uniquely modern demands of industrialization and urbanization (Goddard 1914, 2). In other words, "disability" is not just another word for "social crisis" in all historical contexts; the United States and parts of Europe manufactured the need to constitute a class of disabled citizens when individuals came to be increasingly defined by industrial labor practices within a capitalist marketplace. The demand was *not* one of increasing proficiency, higher levels of training, and the need for a more sophisticated citizenry to embrace a national destiny—although all of these reasons are cited in the literature we discuss. Rather, as we argue in chapter 1 on charity, disability categories proliferate as an increasing value is placed upon bodily homogeneity, concepts of quantifiable health measurement, and the workplace standardization of capacities. It is the product of a nineteenth- and early twentieth-century arsenal that sought to make myriad forms of abnormality visible through the development of disciplines and professions that depend on discovering increasing degrees of human deviance.

The point is more than just a contention that difference comes to be devalued in modernity. Rather, it is that disabled bodies are constituted as unduly discordant within a rapidly solidifying fiction of an idealized American body politic. There was the material body of the citizen (with all of its variety of appearances, capacities, and vulnerabilities) and then there was the idealized body of the nation (with all of its nationalistic implications that propelled the question of individual biology into a matter of public hygiene management). The two "bodies" were intimately conjoined during the period under discussion in this book. No longer were citizens cajoled to take care of themselves for their own well-being and that of their family and immediate neighbors; rather, they came to be increasingly articulated as possessions of the state. To take care of oneself became synonymous with an obligation to the improvement of the nation (Jakubowicz and Meekosha 2002, 2). If the national body was made up of a multitude of individual bodies, then each "person" was recognized as a microcosm of the state.

The transmission of one's hereditary (and later, genetic) material comes to the foreground during this period as the concern of national and state governments, organizations, and state-sponsored science. For the national body to become increasingly "coherent," citizens must begin to recognize themselves as either contributors to or detractors from the overall health of the body politic. The period under scrutiny in this study evolves (or devolves) a perspective on the body that increasingly recognizes biology as the *matter* of the state. Thus, disability comes to be policed in increasingly severe ways, since the only "capital" disabled people are presumed to possess is a set of biological coordinates that must be kept from dissemination within the larger, and more significant, body of the nation (the sum of its generational inheritance).

During this period, which runs roughly from the Jacksonian to the progressive era and beyond, citizens were called upon with increasing frequency to police their own reproductive participation. Thus, eugenics can be comfortably situated alongside a host of other reform movements that took shape during this period. For instance, in the rereleased public health propaganda film, *Are You Fit to Marry?* (originally titled *The Black Stork* [1927 (1917)]), the eugenics physician, Dr. Wirth, tells his daughter's suitor, Jack Gaynor, that "as goes its babies, so goes the nation." The explicit equation of hardy babies with national robustness shows how eugenics promoted the notion that individual bodies stood for national power and purity. Disability was gradually transformed from a private family/community affair where bodies broke down, took sick, evidenced human vulnerability and the interdependency of human lives, into a national scourge that must be sequestered and ultimately ousted from a shared hereditary pool called the "national stock." Building on theories translated from applications of statistical averages, Galton's theories of controlled breeding practices, and Mendelian theories of dominant and recessive gene transmission applied to human communities, eugenicists viewed traits recognized as detrimentally deviant as identifiable, predictable, and therefore, *preventable*. In doing so, disability moved from its characterization in the seventeenth and eighteenth centuries as a matter of exotic monstrosity or personal misfortune to an array of eradicable conditions that, as the prologue of the 1932 release of the movie *Freaks* announces, "will soon be eradicated from the Earth by advances in modern Teratology."

THE END OF DISABILITY   The first half of the twentieth century was consistently characterized as an age when the eradication of disability was within the country's grasp. Such beliefs need to be understood in the context of developments in evolutionary theory and the process by which "defective" human bodies were produced in the wake of Darwin's revolutionary notions of natural selection. Darwin's theory of species adaptation and diversification rested on three key principles, which have great interest for disability studies: (1) all structures vary and therefore evolve; (2) adaptation is random and gradual in nature; (3) fortuitous variations are unpredictable given that shifting environments alone determine organismic viability. As an important aside, Darwin generally distrusted the efficacy of human interventions to control the process and direction of species variation: "How fleeting are the wishes and efforts of man! How short his time! And consequently how poor will his products be" (quoted in Gould 2002, 157).

Opposed to Darwinism were the saltationists. Those who espoused saltationist theories, among whom Sir Francis Galton was the best known, argued against the validity of Darwinian natural selection, based on limitations ("structural constraints") inherent in the germ plasm of organisms. Saltationists argued that species differentiation occurs according to the laws of regression toward the mean, where atypical features, both desirable and undesirable (for example, genius and idiocy), tend to give way to the overreplication of traits considered average or typical across a species. Within this formula saltationist science argued that mean values associated with bodily traits and capacities could be shifted by the adoption of strenuous breeding practices that would encourage desirable characteristics while discouraging undesirable qualities. As Galton put it in his *Hereditary Genius*, published in 1869:

> I propose to show in this book that a man's natural abilities are derived by inheritance, under exactly the same limitations as are the form and physical features of the whole organic world. Consequently, as it is easy, notwithstanding those limitations, to obtain by careful selection a permanent breed of dogs or horses gifted with peculiar powers of running, or of doing anything else, so it would be quite practicable to produce a highly-gifted race of men by judicious marriages during several consecutive generations. I shall show that social agencies of an ordinary character, whose influences are little suspected, are at this moment working towards the degradation of human nature, and that others are working towards its improvement. I conclude that each generation has enormous power over the natural gifts of those that follow, and maintain that it is a duty we owe to humanity to investigate the range of that power, and to exercise it in a way that, without being unwise towards ourselves, shall be most advantageous to future inhabitants of the earth. (2001 [1869], 45)

Unlike Quetelet, the French statistician who, as Lennard Davis has shown (1995), viewed average characteristics as most desirable, Galton was fascinated by extreme points of deviation from the mean. By dismissing the critical principle of Darwinian gradualism as too slow and inefficient to adequately explain species development and differentiation, the eugenicists advocated directed breeding practices. Unlike Darwin, who argued for an

Adam Smith–like, laissez-faire attitude toward adaptation in *On the Origin of Species*, eugenicists (some of whom espoused Darwinist models of evolution) encouraged the practical and overly simplistic application of Mendelian principles to the state oversight of human reproduction (Gould 2002, 122). Eugenics promoted the adoption of public policies that would assure the transfer of desirable characteristics (genius, tall stature, blue eye color, and other features primarily associated with Nordic European peoples) and would discourage the passage of undesirable traits (feeblemindedness, epilepsy, blindness, deafness, congenital impairments, alcoholism, promiscuity, and so forth). Within this scheme of dividing human variations into binary systems of normal and feebleminded, eugenicists encouraged direct intervention in the process of species evolution in order to cultivate some traits at the expense of others in a nation's collective germ plasm.

While the application of horticultural and animal husbandry strategies does not fully account for the development of beliefs about disability that took shape at the beginning of the twentieth century, it laid a foundation stone in the edifice of eugenics proper as it came to be practiced in the United States and much of Europe. One of the misperceptions that we seek to correct in this book is a historical revisionism that characterizes eugenics as a momentary aberration in the history of disability science. Even the late Stephen J. Gould's renowned work on eugenics, *The Mismeasure of Man* (1996 [1981]), encourages a treatment of eugenic science as an aberration of sound empirical practice (see chapter 2, below). More recently, publications sponsored by the Human Genome Project, such as Elof Axel Carlson's *The Unfit: A History of a Bad Idea* (2001), seek to critique eugenics as bad science and in doing so, to place as much distance as possible between its practices and those of contemporary genetics. By marginalizing eugenics in this manner, we risk forgetting or diminishing widespread professional participation in a disgraceful historical chapter. This approach neglects the broader ramifications of a history that continues to have profound implications for the treatment of disabled people in the United States. Such analyses treat eugenics as little more than an inconsequential mutant organism that ultimately proved unviable.

Consequently, the analysis of eugenics practices and beliefs forms the backdrop for the historical drama of disability. We situate eugenics as the centerpiece of U.S. attitudes toward bodies marked as deviant from the mid-nineteenth century to the end of World War II. We also attempt to show how such beliefs developed out of shifts in charity practices and attitudes toward

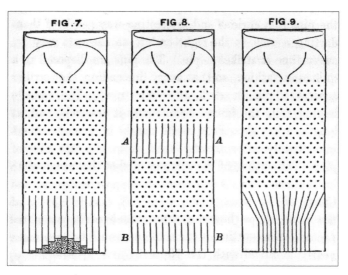

FRANCIS GALTON'S DRAWING OF THE QUIN-CUNX TO DEMONSTRATE HIS CONCEPT
OF STANDARD DEVIATION (BELL CURVE DISTRIBUTIONS). GRAVITY DRAWS PELLETS
THROUGH THE PYRAMIDAL STRUCTURE OF PEGS, WHICH COLLECT AT POINTS A
AND B. FIGURES 7, 8, AND 9 REPRESENT DIFFERENT VERSIONS OF THE MACHINE.
(FROM GALTON 1988 [1889], 63)

disabled beggars, as diagnosed in Herman Melville's novel *The Confidence-Man* (1984 [1857]), and how they have reverberated beyond the two world wars in the institutional treatment of people with "multi-handicaps," such as those depicted in Fred Wiseman's documentary films. Thus, the book pursues readings of scientific and state-authored documents on disability research between analyses of cultural texts. The period of U.S. history represented by these works is, with respect to people with disabilities, the most dynamic and portentous period, which saw the development of an increasingly hostile and restrictive social context for all marginalized populations. In presenting it, we hope to forward some key characteristics of a history of intolerance that can then be more readily detected and dismantled in the years to come.

For example, in the widely studied textbook *Anomalies and Curiosities of Medicine* by George Gould and Walter Pyle (1901), students and practitioners of medicine at the beginning of the twentieth century could scan a veritable freak show of disabled bodies placed on display in medical photographs and illustrations. The collection's subtitle speaks volumes as to the reigning attitude in the medical industries of London, Philadelphia, and Paris with respect to anomalous bodies: "being an encyclopedic collection of rare and extraordinary cases, and of the most striking instances of abnormality in all branches of medicine and surgery, derived from an exhaustive research of medical literature from its origins to the present day, abstracted, classified, annotated and indexed." The work, in other words, participates in a long-standing medical tradition that sought to collect and "preserve" examples of what the sixteenth-century Italian philosopher Fortunio Liceto referred to as *"monstrorum natura caussis"* (1634). For Gould and Pyle, this tradition of medical spectacle based on the display of bodies assigned to the category of the "abnormal" came about when "man's mind first busied itself with subjects beyond his own self-preservation and the satisfaction of his bodily appetites" (ibid., 1). The suggestion here is that alleviation from concern with satisfying basic human needs (a goal that was far from accomplished in the era of industrialization about which this book was written) provided the freedom for more frivolous or dire occupations. Thus, disability comes to be galvanized as a category of investigation into the "anomalous and curious" at the origins of nineteenth-century scientific investigation. It became a sort of pastime for those who had significant professional and leisure time to pursue those others who occupied bodies that suggested the need for the containment of "deviance."

At least in the United States, formal eugenics developed most vigorously during the period from the end of the Civil War to the beginning of World War II. Published in the era of the first theories of heredity, *Anomalies and Curiosities of Medicine* mixes the categories of congenital and environmentally produced differences in a way that mirrors eugenic confusion about whether noncongenital conditions (termed "defects"), such as alcoholism, acquired psychiatric conditions, or the accidental loss of a limb, could be passed on to later generations (questions that in some cases are still being debated today). Research into the origins and consequences of disabilities during this period suggests the degree to which branches of medical and scientific study continue to treat disability paradoxically as both an insoluble mystery and a preoccupation that promises to yield knowledge about nondisabled bodies. This dual structure of disability inquiry pervades the literature and participates in turning disabled people into objects of rampant speculation and a wellspring of medical knowledge of all bodies. Here is a crucial point: *the exhaustion of disabled research subjects comes by way of our historical investment in believing that disability makes a person available for excessive experimentation and bureaucratic oversight.* In this book we seek to identify the eugenic origins of such practices and to trace them as a primary source of disabled

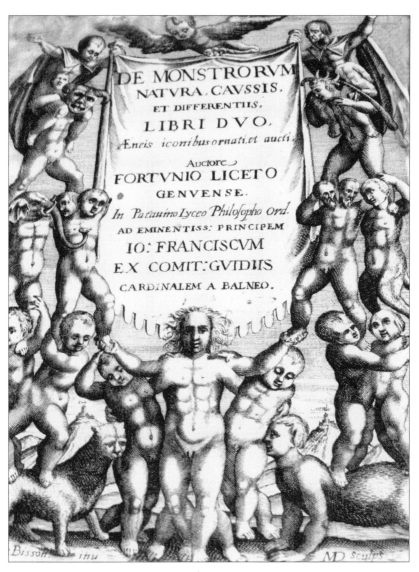

TITLE PAGE OF FORTUNIO LICETO'S «DE MONSTRORUM CAUSSIS, NATURA,
ET DIFFERENTIIS» (1634)

people's oppression today. From this perspective, research feeds the insatiable gristmill of science while also fortifying our ideas of disability as a curiosity that invites the most prurient forms of speculation parading as empiricism.

Not only is this history precipitated by beliefs produced within research science, it also infiltrates mainstream culture. When we speak of the devastating impact of eugenic beliefs, we must also come to terms with the rise of commodification strategies. Eugenics was not only discussed and promoted in scientific journals and eclectic professional publications, it also spread into mass culture in the form of product promotion. The effort to link an image of the idealized national body with mass-marketed products staked a significant claim on investments in a purified race of people rapidly coming to be recognized as "American." The sociologist Paul Gilroy calls this process "logo-solidarity." Adorning products of all kinds were legions of chubby white baby faces and athletic specimens from the physical culture craze of the early twentieth century (2001, 162). These images of Caucasian wholesomeness functioned at all levels of mass-market culture as signs of racial purity and idealized national body types free of blemishes, defects, variations, or vulnerabilities that marked the bodies of consumers themselves. From soap to salt, one purchased not only products, but also a prototypical image of the body that served as a representative for those who could claim a particular belongingness based upon shared features and "biological" qualities. What Foucault calls a "capillary distribution of power" is at work in this formula, in which individual bodies come to be policed through consumption practices at the most infinitesimal levels of culture (1995, 198). Principles of positive eugenics—or the cultivation of public schemes promoting "fitter" families and individuals—become translated into successful marketing strategies. As disabled people find themselves institutionalized in greater numbers, disability is supplanted from public visibility by a market that thrives upon icons of the healthy and wholesome.

This period sees the convergence of public hygiene management schemes, interchangeability of laboring bodies, theories of heredity that led to a discourse of prevention, racialization of national types, fears of unchecked feminine sexuality, and commodification of an increasingly narrow bodily aesthetic. The result is the creation of a lethal social atmosphere. So-called ugly laws (first adopted in the 1880s), marriage laws, coerced institutionalization, and involuntary sterilization all arrived on the dockets of state legislatures as the political expression of increasing cultural intolerance for human differences. By 1914 university researchers Stevenson Smith, Madge Wilkinson, and Louisa Wagoner, on behalf of the Bailey and Babette Gatzert Foundation for Child Welfare, reported that nearly every state in the nation had made it illegal for feebleminded and insane people to marry (566–71), and twenty-five states had involuntary commitment laws (603–4). According to Chicago-based eugenicist Harry Laughlin, by 1922 fifteen states (Washington, California, Connecticut, Indiana, Iowa, New York, New Jersey, Michigan, Kansas, Wisconsin, Nebraska, Nevada, Oregon, North Dakota, and South Dakota) had passed laws permitting coerced sterilization of "the unfit" to prevent the transmission of "defects" from one generation to another (Laughlin 1922, 14). As Edwin Black argues in *War against the Weak*, "because eugenics was administered on the local level, every state probably possesses three to five sites hosting important eugenic documentation" (2003, xix). Many of the remaining states had not yet introduced or acted on sterilization legislation. The widespread adoption of these discriminatory legal and policy efforts forms part of what Zygmunt Bauman (2001b) has identified as the increasingly bureaucratic oversight of lives during modernity.

CONCLUSION: MODERNITY AND DISABILITY   For Bauman, modernity comes packaged according to its foremost theorists, such as Max Weber, as a period of increasing investments in the systematic control of social relations. Within this scenario we witness the triumph of the rational spirit, principles of efficiency, and scientific management, and the relegation of social values to the relativist domain of subjectivity. Among these precepts of modernity (and Bauman does not refute these) one finds the valorization of accomplishment with less expenditure—of energy, of resources, of moral anguish, of human labor. Modernity gives birth to the culture of technology that promises more data from less input. This unique historical terrain is characterized by Bauman as "the morally elevating story of humanity emerging from pre-social barbarity" (2001b, 12). This progressive narrative is key to the development of disability as a concept of deviant variation. In a culture that endlessly assures itself that it is on the verge of conquering Nature once and for all, along with its own "primitive" instincts and the persistent domain of the have-nots, disability is referenced with respect to these idealized visions. As a vector of human variability, disabled bodies both represent a throwback to human prehistory and serve as the barometer of a future without "deviancy."

In other words, for modernity, the eradication of disability represented a scourge and a promise: its presence signaled a debauched present of cultural degeneration that was tending to regress toward a prior state of primitivism, while at the same time it seemed to promise that its absence would mark the completion of modernity as a cultural project. The eradication of disability would be the sign of arrival at a long-sought destination. These predictions were always made within a rhetoric of benign outcomes. Yet those who anticipated the ultimate arrival at a disability-free moment inevitably flirted with the more sinister language of extermination. This analysis falls in line with Bauman's provocative contention that "the Holocaust [was] a 'paradigm' of modern civilization, its 'natural,' its 'normal' (who knows—perhaps *also* common) product, its 'historical tendency'" (2001b, 6). Rather than accept the common sociological argument that the Holocaust was an aberration of the period, an absolutely deviant outcome of an era that aimed to roll back any such impulse in human behavior, Bauman argues that the defining features of technological and bureaucratic genocide were part and parcel of an age obsessed with administrative tidiness. His careful choice of terms here—"natural," "normal," "common"—characterize a European and American cultural mindset that presided over the transition of biologically based differences into pathological social deviancies.

In *Modernity and the Holocaust*, Bauman recognizes modernity as a type of bureaucratic nightmare from which we cannot awake. He contends that treating the Holocaust as a uniquely pathological, extraordinarily brutal event runs the risk of asking nothing of modernity itself or its residents. If we fail to recognize the Holocaust as a byproduct of modern utopian fantasies, then we avoid the task of making urgent critiques of our own fetishization of normativity as the outcome of a narrow, homogeneous social vision. As we discuss in chapter 3, the feasibility of mass murder and the development of genocidal killing technologies in Nazi Germany were all perfected on the bodies of disabled people in preparation for the Holocaust. This historical recognition asks us to contemplate more earnestly the degree to which the eradication of disability *and* the Holocaust are "part and parcel" of modernity. There is something materially stubborn about bodies in this period that precipitate so many disastrously "plausible" radical solutions in their name. The body becomes not just a site of social regulation but also a location of excesses and insufficiencies—what is referred to as "too much and too little of a body." The "practicality" of Nazi extermination came about after assiduous study of the problems of human remains disposal; burning those murdered in crematoria ovens was a way of further destroying the recalcitrant biological remainder left over from the killing programs. It was the ultimate fantasy of invisibility.

On the way to this desecration of bodies, modernity, according to Bauman, undertakes three distinct operations with respect to an adequate lessening of moral inhibitions: "And so, how were these ordinary Germans transformed into the German perpetrators of mass crime? In the opinion of Herbert C. Kelman, moral inhibitions against violent atrocities tend to be eroded once three conditions are met, singly or together; the violence is *authorized* (by official orders coming from the legally entitled quarters), actions are *routinized* (by rule governed practices and exact specification of roles), and the victims of violence are *dehumanized* (by ideological definitions and indoctrinations)" (2001b, 21). This is the exact recipe of eugenics with respect to the treatment of disability. State policies were passed that barred people with disabilities from social participation. Confinement, away from the mainstream, was commonly implemented upon those whose bodies existed outside of acceptable bodily norms and aesthetics. Eugenicists openly and excessively degraded their clientele in their professional rhetoric of "objectivity." We would only add to this list a growing hostility toward the "mean" characteristics (that is, routine instances of biological diversity) of a population. Together, these conditions provide the foundations for a eugenics culture. Identifying them allows us to assess the extent to which our own era replicates an ideology of extinction disguised beneath rhetorics of assistance, support, and cure.

We have written this book for at least four different audiences at the same time. For students and scholars in history and disability studies, the sites examined offer important examples of the formative interactions between the emergent category of disability and the systems among which it was forged. The development of this institutional history allows one to get a better grasp on the cultural roles played by disability and the degree to which disability, as a profoundly marginalized social grouping, manages to function as a critical term in U.S. and Western definitions of embodiment.

For administrators, researchers, and advocates of disability (largely outside of disability studies proper), this book seeks to provide a series of cautions about ethical imperatives surrounding any study of disability. What we hope becomes most evident in this history is how violent exclusions are enacted in the name of benign (and even radically political) practices toward disabled people. To this end, we identify an intellectual genealogy of disability in the nineteenth and twentieth centuries in a way that has not been presented before (with the exception, perhaps, of James Trent's important work, *Inventing the Feeble Mind: A History of Mental Retardation in the United States* [1994]). We also criticize—in the hopes of inciting more discussion— the degree to which disabled persons–based research can be useful at all. This last point is our most controversial argument, as we stress an overall, cumulative exhaustion of research practices upon disabled citizens since the mid-nineteenth century. Even the contemporary academy continues to pursue "more research on disability" with unquestioned assumptions about the ethics of the perpetual availability of disabled bodies.

We have also tried to address a general readership, for whom the ideas discussed in this work prove both disturbing and compelling as one tries to reconstruct the history of current beliefs about disability. Unlike the authors of much current research based on disability and disability studies, we have taken it for granted that one cannot adequately assess any object without knowing its particular (and often peculiar) origins. Disability plays a critical role in how we formulate relationships between ourselves and others—all of them connected to Western concepts of difference, variation, and the meaning of human deviation.

Lastly, we write for readers who themselves might be disabled or actively involved in disability activist movements in the United States and internationally. For those readers, this work forwards an argument not just about U.S. and Western beliefs about disability, but also about the power and volume of written and spoken discourse about this object of research. We would like readers to come away from this study not just with a sense of the dehumanizing networks of beliefs that exist about disability and disabled people, but also with an understanding that disability research is about the historical effort to concretize cultural fantasies about "biological" difference. In this respect, our hope is to make evident the formal structures at work in bringing disability into direct relationship with a form of subhumanity—a process that further entrenches disabled people in this cultural location of disability while continually acting as if the ultimate goal is our rescue from this debased placement.

Part I

DIS-LOCATIONS

OF

CULTURE

ONE

Masquerades of Impairment

Charity as a Confidence Game

SURFACE SCIENCES The nineteenth century oversaw a transition from practices of community responsibility for poverty and disability. An increasingly centralized, national economy gave rise to intrusive managerial attitudes toward pauperism and diverse human capacities and appearances. The seventeenth and early eighteenth centuries had tended to approach human differences from a religious standpoint of the "strong" taking care of the "weak." In contrast, the nineteenth century approached dependency as a disservice to a nation that must invest in its manifest destiny. Jacksonian America provided an important venue for practices founded on physical observation: craniometry, phrenology, palmistry, psychology, and physiognomy (Otter 1999). Each investigative field sought a passage into the intangible interior of human personality through the body as its signifying medium. The psychic constitution of individuals could be accessed through careful scrutiny of anatomy as a mirror to otherwise invisible phenomena. Thus, human bodies—particularly those marked as "crippled" or "queer" or "deviant"—supported efforts to delineate between deserving and undeserving poor as proper recipients of public and private philanthropic initiatives.

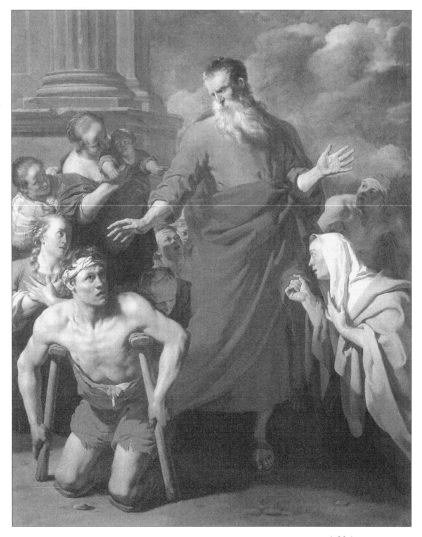

KAREL DUJARDIN, «ST. PAUL HEALING THE CRIPPLE AT LYSTRA» (1663)

These "sciences of the surface" were based on the belief that external body features functioned as reliable markers by which the identity of a person could be fixed. Embodiment increasingly came to adjudicate a person's social worth. In this respect, U.S. responses to physical, sensory, and cognitive impairments (actual and perceived, functional and aesthetic) changed from a relatively benign formula, the interdependency of human lives in an immediate community, to one of moral judgment practiced in many American communities.¹ Those classified as economically dependent—because they could not participate in rigid social roles without significant revision to modes of work, habitat, and socialization rituals—often became pariahs. Families came to be held culpable for the unpreparedness of their members for vigorous national participation—particularly with respect to employability. Furthermore, charity discourses of this period often held out faulty lifestyles as the source of impairments, finding both families and individuals culpable for manifestations of specific bodily and cognitive anomalies.

While the later science of eugenics deepened the reliance on the body as an external manifestation of malignant psychic structures, this period in American history is the first to introduce disability as disruptive to rationales of national citizenship. Disability precluded one's right to access modes of civic belonging that granted social privileges. Because disability came to be construed as a fully tragic consequence of embodiment gone awry, one that extracted individuals from productive membership in a capitalist economy, people with physical and cognitive differences found themselves controlled by new terms: those of the emergent modern charity concepts of the industrial United States. Disabled people found that their livelihood and integration were no longer perceived as a matter of familial and community responsibility; instead, they were to be officially classified by scientific techniques adopted for producing objectifying taxonomies of the body. Named as members of a deficient population—the legion of the defective, delinquent, nonproductive, and the burdensome—disabled bodies increasingly came to be managed by private organizations as well as state and federal agencies. This process of cultural dislocation marks a critical moment in American approaches to disability and the rise of pervasive bodily detection strategies required for charity oversight as an extension of newly professionalizing medical authority.

DISABILITY AS DEPENDENCY Often individuals with disabilities in need of "public assistance" due to lack of economic opportunity were labeled as "dependent." Like slaves and indentured servants, disabled people occupied roles as vagrants ruled incapable of entering into voluntary contracts of labor as a result of dependency. As Eric Foner argues, this intolerance for dependency was inherited from the previous century: "it was an axiom of eighteenth-century political thought that dependents lacked a will of their own, and thus did not deserve a role in public affairs" (1995, xii). Yet, while many social historians have found the classification of dependency to be peopled in primarily "racial terms" (Foner 1995, xxvii), others have recognized the class of beggars as representing a wider cultural cross-section of labor refugees who were not allowed "into the matrix of contract relations" (Stanley 1998, xiii). In fact, the definition of beggars and other social unfortunates of this time became synonymous with social irresponsibility and willed incapacity, as their presumed unsuitability for labor was a choice rather than a socially conditioned fate: "The beggar was the most conspicuous figure of dependency and, in [nineteenth-century] opinion, the most loathsome—a suspect figure who allegedly thrived on deception rather than work, someone who got something for nothing. . . . Supposedly, the beggar only pretended to seek work, 'coining his unblushing falsehoods as fast as he can talk,' while violating the divine rule of labor that charity agencies took as their watchword: 'He that will not work, neither shall he eat' " (Stanley 1998, 103). As Michael J. Sandel points out, this analysis of beggars mirrored arguments against the wealthy classes whom Jacksonians referred to as "nonproducers" and as those who benefited most from a market economy but "contributed least" (1996, 154). Such suspicions of purposeful parasitism on the part of beggars show that most laboring people under capitalism were never far from poverty themselves.

The charity industries hailed from an increasingly outdated ethos of paternal relations. The rigors of a market exchange economy had come to dominate the period, and charity struck many people as a social throwback to the days of colonial protectionism and dependency. Charity was fully part of an exchange-based economy; it performed a crucial oversight task by ensuring that those who did not work were not enticed by the "ease of pauperism." One had to give up something to receive social aid, and what one "exchanged" were the liberties that presumably constituted the "inalienable" rights of citizens. Charity stepped in to assure everyone that a life of poverty was simultaneously "deserved" and necessarily untenable.

At the same time, charity reformers of this period advocated laws that removed begging from public view. Rather than indicting an inflexible and unequal system of contract labor, charity officials demanded, with local police and in the courts, the criminalization of individuals reduced to begging. Passage of the 1834 New Poor Law, harsh antivagrancy laws, and "tramp" acts or vagabond laws in cities across the country essentially made it a crime to beg openly in the streets (Stanley 1998, 112–13). Imprisonment, forced labor, and expulsion awaited those arrested for "alms crying." The responsibility for the violation of such statutes was not upon those who gave alms, but rather upon those who made the request. Thus, simply asking for alms became illegal in many parts of the country. In criminalizing begging, the legislatures drew

40

a connection between beggar and criminal. Both, after all, sought to take something for nothing. Thus, they threatened a system of exchange by refusing to comply with one of its foundational premises. The class consternation over "refusals to work" on the part of "sturdy beggars" and the privilege of getting something for nothing on the part of "cripples and other unfortunates" led to the institution of workhouses and other modes of enforced labor originally used in Europe to extract class compliance. Thus, charity in this period was transformed from a matter of paternal relations into a system in which those who received handouts increasingly found themselves punished for their need (Stanley 1998, 135).

Widespread class anxieties over the precariousness of capitalist relations led to the cultivation of an apparatus to anticipate who was likely to become a public "burden." The system relied on methodologies forwarded by "sciences of the surface." Its operations can be seen in the passage of severe immigration restrictions on those with physical or mental impairments; antivagrancy ordinances and "tramp laws" that denied a town's obligation to help those who arrived impoverished from other areas; and "ugly laws" that banned physical "unsightliness" from appearances in public areas. As the ugly laws show, these systems of anticipatory classification were often based on bodily aesthetics rather than literal abilities. Physiognomic practices became a staple of the new "science of alms" and played a key role in an era that judged itself proficient at assessing citizens' worth on the basis of their possession of a full range of normative bodily, sensory, and cognitive capacities. In many cases the exclusion of those with disabilities was based on the desire of manufacturers to employ workers without need for modification of labor conditions.

For those who fell short of this labor expectation, charity organizations assured that "excessive" need could be met with stern disapproval, moral disapprobation, and patronizing religious instruction. At the same time charity also provided a public benefit in recognizing individual contribution as a sign of beneficence, generosity, and commitment to capitalist values of self-reliance. Charity's provision of such an outlet for moralistic example demonstrates what disability historian Paul Longmore defines as the practice of conspicuous contribution: a cultural ritual in which the "economically able" garishly donate in public venues to help disabled people and bolster their own renown (1997, 146). Within these economic rituals, "disability" itself becomes a matter of performative interdependency as disabled bodies are made to appear unduly dependent and donors further solidify their own social value as able benefactors.

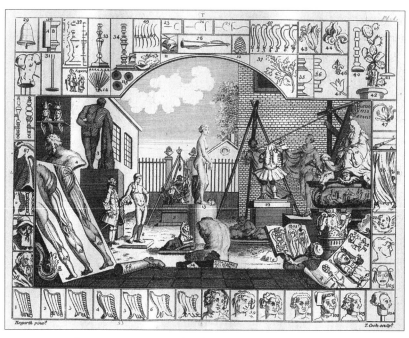

HOGARTH'S «ANALYSIS OF BEAUTY» (1753) APPLIED PHYSIOGNOMIC PRINCIPLES OF
APPEARANCE TO IMAGES OF STANDARD BEAUTY. (FROM «HOGARTH'S WORKS,» 2 VOLS.
[LONDON: LEWIS AND COMPANY, 1804], 2:105)

Accounts by social historians of the rise of this new U.S. charity system have provided important analyses of this period's practices and attitudes toward charity. Little attention has been paid, however, to the fate of those impoverished as a result of physical and cognitive impairments (congenital or acquired). This is true even among those historians who recognize the class of beggars as a diverse, disenfranchised social constituency. One commentator who did take up a socioeconomic approach to disability and alms-seeking was the mid-nineteenth-century American writer, Herman Melville. For Melville, the cultural obsession with the "sturdy beggar" subjected all alms-seekers to the test of the distinction between the deserving and undeserving poor; however, in the case of beggars made unemployable by disability—we guess this would make them "unsturdy beggars"—begging itself was elevated to the level of performance art. Thus, the confidence games that take place aboard the steamship *Fidèle* in his book *The Confidence-Man: His Masquerade* (published in 1857) depend upon a level of sophisticated deception—even art. Disabled people are recognized as those who must adeptly manipulate suspicious and surly social belief systems about their potential masquerades of incapacity and their parasitism. Nineteenth-century capitalism thus produced disabled people as ever-visible actors on a debasing stage. Their definitive parasitism is both publicly chastened and embraced as a welcome distraction from the inequalities of a newly solidifying, exchange-based economy. Disabled people functioned as a warning of the instability of capitalism and as an assurance to "normal" people that their own situation was better than that of many.

Melville's entrance into debates over impairment and vagrancy hinges on four distinct critiques relevant to the cultural production of disabled bodies during this time: (1) through the conflation of charity solicitations and confidence games as activities that connected economic behavior with moral action; (2) as a critique of charity systems that excluded recipients from robust participation as national citizens; (3) as an exposé of capitalist altruism that markets products and services through opportune references to the alleviation of human suffering; and (4) as narrative device, powerful because of its ability to function as spectacle, and hence available to unmoor concepts of fixed orders and roles. Our opening analysis focuses on the first of these critiques, exposing the inequitable power relations at work in nineteenth-century U.S. capitalism. Melville's representation of disabled bodies in *The Confidence-Man* serves as a basis for delineating an economics of anatomy, charity, and social role already operating in this period; the attendant cultural displacement that accompanied stigmatized biological differences offers a stepping-stone to the cultural location of disability in nineteenth-century U.S. culture.

DISABILITY AND THE MATERIALITY OF THE SIGN

The Confidence-Man wages warfare on "sciences of the surface" for presuming, on behalf of scientific and national knowledge, the reliability of bodily appearance as a means to evaluate the social worth of persons. In doing so, Melville's narrative returns to a critique of the cultural practices that the narrating Ishmael had dismissed in *Moby-Dick* as "semi-sciences" and "passing fables," in order to interrogate the use of assessments of physicality in making moral appraisals and economic decisions.[2] Melville takes up these critiques of visual assessment practices to foreground the deceptions of bodies, and to evaluate capitalist charity exchanges that not only support, but also produce, socially inequitable bodies.

The Confidence-Man interrogates scientific and charity efforts to make disability function as a reliable sign of human depravity. This strategy of remarking on human "grotesqueries" was relatively new in the period, for

43

never before had disability achieved the full status of a discernible "needy" constituency in the United States. In his 1848 report to the Massachusetts legislature on the newly minted condition of "idiocy," Samuel Gridley Howe, then director of what would become the Perkins Institute for the Blind, petitioned for an endowment that would allow the establishment of the first training school in the United States on behalf of "idiots." Following the practices of Itard and Séguin that he witnessed in France, Howe defined "idiocy" as a diagnostic classification of "sufferers . . . found in a degree of physical deterioration, and of mental and moral darkness" (Howe 1848, 29). Such embodied conditions identify a new industry of disability, one that promotes the necessity of undertaking research on a previously neglected population for "[e]vils cannot be grappled with, and overcome, unless their nature and extent are fully known" (Howe 1848, 29).

Within this scenario legislatures should give researchers the funding (a form of scientific charity) to compile empirical evidence on various aspects of "bodily organization" that will inevitably come to be recognized in the future as the root cause of human deficiency:

> The whole subject of idiocy is new. Science has not yet thrown her certain light upon its remote, or even its proximate causes. There is little doubt, however, that they are to be found in the CONDITION OF THE BODILY ORGANIZATION. The size and shape of the head, therefore; the proportionate development of its different parts; the condition of the nervous system; the temperament; the activity of the various functions; the development of the great cavities;—the chest and abdomen; the stature,—the weight,—every peculiarity, in short, that can be noted in a great number of individuals, may be valuable to future observers. We contribute our own observations to the store of facts, out of which science may, by and by, deduce general laws. If any bodily peculiarities, however minute, always accompany peculiar mental conditions, they become important; they are the finger-marks of the Creator, by which we learn to read his works. (Howe 1848, 31)

Unlike their French counterparts, U.S. investigators of idiocy placed great emphasis on surface physical qualities as the route to an enlightened knowledge of "peculiar mental conditions." The body is transformed into a yet-to-be-explored topography, whose inner secrets will be revealed. Here we can recognize the first stirrings of eugenic philosophy in the United States. In Howe's view, the promise of knowledge about human differences will not only teach audiences the value of scientific inquiry, but also give them tangible evidence of the workings of a divine creator whose behind-the-scenes handiwork is evident in the trace, or "finger-marks," that remain legible upon the sculpted surface of humanity. Disabled people are thus tantamount to imperfect vessels formed by the fingers of an unskilled potter.

Such investigations of idiocy situate the nineteenth century on the cusp of a social transition from religious to scientific interpretive frameworks. Disability is central to this enterprise in that its status as the most visible sign of "human degeneracy" promises to offer something in exchange to otherwise competing social systems of explanation. Correlations between physical and cognitive anomalies underwrite the legitimacy of "sciences of the surface" and also offer an empirical method for differentiating among various categories of human beings—particularly those in need of moral and bodily uplift.

Such is the backdrop for *The Confidence-Man*. To capture the array of pejorative beliefs that disability spawned in the nineteenth century, Melville's tale begins with a rare scene in narrative literature: an array of disabled characters occupying a shared social space. In part, this unusual gathering of "misfits" resulted from increasing public concern over the "swelling ranks" of impoverished people who began to appear on street corners and form lines at soup kitchens (Stanley 1998, 102). These groups of paupers were made up not only of unemployed "common laborers and domestic servants," but also of those who had been ousted from the competitive labor market as a result of impairment. Melville remarks on this new situation of displaced workers throughout the novel, but his particular interest turns to physical and sensory disabilities as the site where one must turn begging into a veritable trade. Denied other options beyond the petty hassles and human diminishment of the organized charity industry, Melville's disabled characters are left to fend for themselves. The art of alms crying serves as the stage upon which disabled people must hone their talents or fall off the social map all together.

At the outset of the novel, the unusual nature of such a gathering of disabled people in public causes the man in the ruby-colored velvet vest to exclaim, "You—pish! Why will the captain suffer these begging fellows on board?" (Melville 1984 [1857], 37). A full-scale assemblage of multiply variant bodies provides Melville with an opportunity to represent disability in a less allegorical manner than in the disabled characters found in many of his other works, such as the prostheticized Ahab or the stammering Billy Budd. The staging of such a multiplicity of disabled characters also provides an unprecedented moment where marked and disqualifying human features demand attention and make disability integral to the mechanism of social interpretation.

The absence of disabled people from the streets and public gathering spaces prior to the nineteenth century turned disability into a rarely encountered phenomenon—at least on a mass scale. This tradition of treating disability as a private family matter functioned as a form of social invisibility; practices of closeting physical, sensory, and cognitive differences within the home made the existence of disability appear less persistent in human communities. Lacking common public venues for interactions with a full range of bodily variability, American culture obscured the necessary demand that communities accommodate multiplicity in the body politic. The relative absence of public disability allows communities to participate in the illusion of social acceptance without contemplating the material and social dynamics by which some people's bodies have been marked as excessive to sustained social policy. Without the necessity of demands on accessible and flexible social environments, disabled people function almost exclusively as a lesson for the nondisabled, promoting behaviors such as patience, cheerfulness, and "making the best of things." These behaviors, as Keith (2001) points out, are also those traditionally taught to women and other social minorities.

In staging a convention of cripples aboard the *Fidèle*, *The Confidence-Man* not only diverges from the traditional portrayal of disability as an individual concern or moral uplift for the nondisabled, it also exposes the dependency of the nation on those defined as biologically inferior. Disabled people represent prototypical nonproducers in exchange economies because the terms of their social participation often exceed a system's willingness to accommodate them. Consequently, disabled people become parasitical, or so runs the narrative of capitalism, and their efforts at subsistence within an exchange-based system offer those recognized as productive participants— a benefactor class—leverage in the social performance of beneficence. *The Confidence-Man* unveils disability's centrality to achieving this goal by examining the degree to which bodies marked as deviant provide an opportunity to solidify other social actors' beliefs in their own moral goodness and proximity to normative ideals. In other words, the benefactor (productive) classes rely on those defined as "nonproductive" to disguise their own economic parasitism on other workers' labor. Through this inversion of social relations, Melville's novel situates the confidence game as that which unveils dependency as a reversible social relation.

To demonstrate dependency as a fluctuating social investment, two discourses compete for attention in *The Confidence-Man*: charity and confidence. The opening chapter situates both terms in proximity to each other in order to anticipate the narrative's argument about their intertwined history. As the passengers embark and gather into various cliques on the ship's topside, a man described as a "Deaf-Mute in cream-colours" holds up a chalk-board exhortation confidently proclaiming charity as a universal good. At the same time a barber opens shop by posting a shingle that declares "No Trust" (the flip side of confidence) to discourage potential clients seeking a haircut on credit. The two signs make competing appeals to the moral and economic instincts of the passengers aboard the *Fidèle*. Yet, while the staging of these two discourses seems antithetical—the former appeals to a biblical good, while the latter refuses all faith in the guarantee of future payment—both signs espouse an absolutist principle for their respective audiences. According to the Deaf-Mute's sign, charity is always a positive virtue, while the barber's capitalist instincts refuse trust in every case. An either/or interpretive system is established, and the story sets out to test both principles as an experiment in the validity of American faith in absolutes.

To draw the terms of charity and confidence into a shared lineage, the third-person narrator points out that the assembled crowd receives each claim in markedly distinct ways. While the Deaf-Mute is jostled and ignored by those passing him, and his multiple disabilities heighten the perception of his "singularity, if not lunacy" (5), the barber's equally "mute" posting elicits no such suspicion. As the narrator explains, the barber's "illuminated paste-board sign" (an intimation of Ahab's reference to the artificiality of paste-board masks in *Moby-Dick*) provokes no "corresponding derision or surprise, much less indignation; and still less, to all appearances, did it gain for the inscriber the repute of being a simpleton" (5). In squaring off these competing systems—the theological against the new science of economy—we see the coming eclipse of religion by economics as a stand-in for a variety of enlightenment-based systems of empiricism. While theologically based beliefs preached tolerance for the less fortunate and thereby often undermined the humanity of the recipient class, the new science of economics evinced a more cut-throat philosophy in which misfortune is a sign of personal insufficiency within a competitive market system. When insufficiency is individualized in this manner, no compensation or accommodation is necessary, for everyone must fend for themselves.

On board the *Fidèle* only the Deaf-Mute's message is greeted with suspicion. People's horror at the revelation that the "man in cream-colours" is "not only dumb but also deaf" transforms him into an object to be shunned. His appearance overrides the content of his message, as the crowd realizes that he is an object of charity and not just an advocate of its virtues: "Meanwhile, he with the slate continued moving slowly up and down, not without causing some stares to change into jeers, and some jeers into pushes, and some pushes into punches" (10). Regardless of the content—one could easily become suspicious of a sign such as "No Trust" as an absolute condition of commerce in a capitalist system—the disabled body plays a key role in the reception of the message, and thus the prime value of charity is excluded, while the prohibition on credit is woven into the fabric of everyday economic relations.

Despite their antithetical receptions both declarations appeal to modes of faith. Neither can secure empirical evidence of its intrinsic value: a divine deity cannot be proven to exist, any more than capital can assert its basis in anything other than symbolic value. This play of surfaces—charity chalkboard and "No Trust" sign—establishes a key conflict that continues through the story. Yet both charity and credit depend upon a future tense of reimbursement for effort. In relation to charity, the bestower will be rewarded in the afterlife, while credit (or trust) will be paid back at a later date for a service delivered in the present. These parallels establish credit and charity as related forces within a market economy, and connect the two terms within a shared cultural genealogy. Their interchange marks the point at which moral and economic systems converge and bolster each other.

Not only does the disabled body draw out suspicions about calls to charity, it also gives rise to social speculation about the meanings ascribed to bodily differences. Once the Deaf-Mute has retired on a vacant ladder to take a nap, the crowd above him begins to speculate on the meaning of his identity. From innocence to monstrosity, each passenger takes a turn at imposing a definition on the Deaf-Mute as a figure of difference. The responses run the full circuit of cultural possibilities for interpreting the disabled body (7): "ODD FISH!" "Who can he be?" "Uncommon countenance." "Green prophet from Utah." "Humbug!" "Singular innocence." "Means something." "Spirit-rapper." "Moon-calf." "Piteous." What bolsters each contention is a belief that deafness and muteness *means something*. The figure's differences—although largely invisible in a physical sense—prompt efforts to interpret a metaphysical principle informing disabled identity. Like the later stories of racial difference in the tales of the Native American termagant, Goneril, and John Mooredock's disquisitions on Indian-hating, disability signals something amiss in the universe, and the onlookers instinctively set about getting to the bottom of the mystery. As Henri-Jacques Stiker argues with respect to the ancient Greeks, the "mystery" of disability is never just a question of how divergent bodies come to be—there is an implication of the entire community in the attribution of difference (1999, 40). It is as if a deviance in the accepted order of things implies that society must master difference in order to turn aside an omen of things to come.

Efforts to define the meaning of the Deaf-Mute's body are unsuccessful. Many of the passengers participate, but no consensus is reached. Instead, the crowd's interpretations collide in an orchestrated multiplicity of beliefs, and the effort to master difference through language is unrealized. The amateur physiognomists on board identify in the sight of the disabled body an opportunity to ply their skills.[3] In doing so, the interpreters all participate in devising a body hierarchy—one that the social construction of disability inaugurates—a form of human objectification based on the interpretation of physical and sensory differences. The Deaf-Mute may be monstrous, naïve, innocent, pitiable, or a Bible-thumper, but all definitions redound to his disadvantage. Once identified as disabled, the Deaf-Mute's figure is quickly transformed into a foreign intruder within their midst; one whose difference threatens to prey on the other passengers' wealth and possibly damage their personal sense of security in their own well-being.

As the passengers expound on the meanings of "the man in cream-colours" to each other, they also solidify their mutual membership in the realm of the normal. The Deaf-Mute's debasement conversely solidifies the crowd's desired proximity to bodily ideals governing questions of social belonging. Thus, while Melville describes the ship's clientele as being a "piebald parliament, an Anacharsis Cloots congress of all kinds of the multiform pilgrim species man" (14), disability involves a degree of difference that cannot be accommodated among even this motley crew. For Melville, the point is not which meaning should be ascribed to the appearance of a disabled body, but rather that the manifestation of disability calls into action an interpretive social mechanism. The disabled characters are disallowed the cover of anonymity on the ship; as the narrator explains, anonymity is a "boon not often withheld from so humble an applicant as [the Deaf-Mute]" (13).

The seemingly sudden appearance of disability in the nineteenth century threatens to disrupt social relations that might otherwise pass as natural and uncorrupted. Just as in *Moby-Dick*, where the *Pequod*'s myriad ethnicities, races, and masculine body types cannot integrate Ahab's prostheticized body successfully into their variegated society, *The Confidence-Man* also holds out disability as an exceptional difference. But while in the former novel, Ahab is condemned to a deterministic existence as a "monomaniacal" disabled man, the latter work undertakes an examination of the inassimilable excess that disability represents to a capitalist order.[4] For instance, while the ship's passengers condemn the man in cream-colours to the stigmatized fate of a deviant species ("ODD FISH!") or to infantilization ("Singular innocence"), the third-person narrator provides an alternative perspective on his figure: "His aspect was at once gentle and jaded, and, from the moment of seating himself, increasing in tired abstraction and dreaminess. Gradually overtaken by slumber, his flaxen head dropped, his whole lamb-like figure relaxed, and, half reclining against the ladder's foot, lay motionless, as some sugar-snow in March, which, softly stealing down over the night, with its white placidity startles the brown farmer peering out from his threshold at daybreak" (11). The image of the placidity of an unexpected snowfall in March and the brown farmer's face peering out onto a landscape transformed at daybreak creates a stunning effect. An unexpected deviation may catch a viewer by surprise, but such a phenomenon does not have to lead the viewer to lessen its power through a defilement of difference. The narrative provides a model by which we might look at variation as something other than symptomatic of disgrace or the need to reinvest ourselves with the superiority gained by an artificially crafted distance from an unexpected phenomenon.

Rather than allow popular discourse to circumscribe the parameters of the "man in cream-colours" as pure deficit, Melville transforms the Deaf-Mute from a threat into the mythic incarnation of a "daylight Endymion" (12). His menacing qualities are emptied out in this description, and the meanings of his differences are inverted into something more akin to a philosopher than a rogue. No longer that of a singular pariah, the figure's appearance allows the narrative to usher in an alternative story in which the reader can recontextualize the figure in a less objectifying manner. Not that his identity is fixed—as Ellen Samuels (2005) points out, the Deaf-Mute's donning of "cream-colours" situates him in a more ambiguous racial and class location than other racially and economically marked characters—rather, the identity of disability is suddenly on the move and can no longer be taken for granted as residing in a static social locale.

The Confidence-Man enacts a developed critique of efforts to make the body into a reliable signifier of a person's humanity. While the "cripples" all come under suspicion in the narrative as either disabled pretenders or human beings unduly soured by their bodily "calamities," the narrator takes up each derogatory dismissal as an opportunity to destabilize the social construction of disability. When the merchant returns to the subject of Black Guinea's miserable life, as evidenced by his "twisted legs" that reduce him to begging, his analysis is exposed as an imposition of his own assumptions rather than a fact of life in a disabled body: "But his companion suggested whether the alleged hardships of that alleged unfortunate might not exist more in the pity of the observer than the experience of the observed" (59). The disjunction between the interpretation of life in a disabled body and the variable experience of lived embodiment provides Melville with the wedge necessary to distance the body from its seemingly stable social meanings. While the disabled body continues to be referenced throughout the narrative as proof of a life unworthy of human dignity, the destabilization of signifier and signified continually threatens to unhinge the visible world from its ideological investments in the depravity of disabled lives. As the "gimlet-eyed," one-legged, "dismissed custom-house officer" knows best of all: "Looks are one thing and facts another" (20). Each opening of the chasm between sign (disability), signifier (pathology), and signified (embodied difference) creates more room for *The Confidence-Man* to perform its interruptive labor upon systems of meaning, a labor that makes the array of cultural signifiers more fluid and less inflexible with respect to their referenced objects.

DISABILITY AND THE ORIGINS OF U.S. CHARITY   While the early chapters of *The Confidence-Man* take up the question of the disabled body as a material index of social station, the majority of the work addresses the charity system's collusion with capitalism in supplying stories of benevolence in an exchange-based economy. For Melville, charity exists as an outpost of inequality for disabled people and/or paupers. As a static signifier of human insufficiency, the disabled body served as one of the foundations on which the nineteenth-century charity system grounded its interventions for the "needy." As many social theorists have pointed out, seventeenth- and eighteenth-century U.S. economic systems approached disability as a familial and communal responsibility that did not require segregation from the social order (Jones 1984, 153–65; Rothman 1971, 319; Trattner 1994, 16–31; Wright 1992, 14–23). Historically, disability has served as a key social category that eminently qualifies an individual for public assistance (along with old age, sickness, and childhood) (Stone 1984, 25). Disabled individuals found themselves exempted from the cultural mandate to work that developed as an essential social expectation of all people during the industrial era.

Charity sought to legislate between a work/need dichotomy by helping to establish reliable classifications of those who deserved assistance as opposed to those drawn toward a life of idleness (Dick 2000, 367; Stone 1984, 54; Waugh 2001, 225). The body became a key adjudicator in debates around poor laws in Europe from the sixteenth century onward (Stone 1984, 30), for instance, because disability seemed to provide a reliable material basis for membership in the need-based classification system: "The [disability] categories solved the work/need dilemma by limiting alms or relief to precisely the people who could not move around anyway: the acutely ill, the physically and mentally disabled, the very old and the very young" (Stone 1984, 54). Within such a system immobility (both biological and culturally imposed) proved critical for deciding who could qualify as a deserving beneficiary of charity and other social assistance schemes.

The Confidence-Man responds to an extensive U.S. tradition of charity as a necessary antidote to the power inequities that accrue in capitalism. We will briefly rehearse this history here in order to establish the historical and cultural bases for Melville's justifiable suspicion of charity as a system that perpetuates, rather than alleviates, social inequality. From the colonial era onward, charity had been promoted as the grease that turns economic divisions between wealthy and poor into a complementary benefit for givers and receivers alike. Although charity evolved over the nineteenth century into an exclusively monetary arrangement between the state and its more dependent citizens during the nineteenth-century, the groundwork for this development was laid in the early colonial period.

For instance, the inaugural sermon delivered by John Winthrop aboard the *Arbella* to the first Puritan immigrants declares that Christian charity will play a critical role in their experimental settlement. Rather than posit equal opportunity for all, Winthrop's sermon argues that charity exists in order "that He might have the more occasion to manifest the work of His Spirit: first upon the wicked in moderating and restraining them, so that the rich and mighty should not eat up the poor, nor the poor and despised rise up against their superiors and shake off their yoke; secondly in the regenerate, in exercising His graces, in them, as in the great ones, their love, mercy, gentleness, temperance, etc.; in the poor and inferior sort, their faith, patience, obedience, etc." (Winthrop 1997, 37). For Winthrop and the Puritans, charity provides an opportunity for wealthy and destitute to participate in a mutually affirming system of economic relations. The "rich and mighty" cultivate qualities such as mercy, gentleness, and temperance toward the socially subordinate, and the "poor and despised" learn to accept such sentiments with faith, patience, and obedience. The wealthy man becomes a paternalistic benefactor while the poor one learns to accept existence on the margins of subsistence with intermittent relief. While social hierarchies are a given, even at the inception of this utopian religious settlement, charity functions as a purifying force that combats moral decay and eases class tensions.

In establishing charity as the cornerstone of religious and economic well-being in the New World, Winthrop draws on a lengthy European tradition of placing benevolence at the nexus between mercantilist and spiritual orders.[5] Charity, Winthrop predicts, will play a critical role in the colony through its ability to unite two distinct economic sectors of civil society: "All men being thus [by divine providence] ranked into two sorts, riche and poore; under the first are comprehended all such as are able to live comfortably by their own meanes duely improved; and all others are poore according to the former distribution . . . as sometimes there may be an occasion of showing mercy to a rich man in some sudden danger or distresse, and alsoe doeing of meere justice to a poor man in regard of some perticular contract" (1997, 38). Within these examples there is an opportunity for each class to perform good works; yet, while the rich may "occasionally" find themselves in physical danger, the poor are marked by their perpetual need of financial relief: "This duty of mercy is exercised in the kinds, giving, lending and forgiving" (ibid.). The "contract" presumes the existence of an economic relationship between the two groups, and consequently, the needs of "riche and poore" converge. A Christian principle of "love towards one's neighbors" promises to secure harmonious economic relations by warding off social discord.

To operate in the interstices of these key social domains, charity played two related roles: as a path to salvation, charity would allow the wealthy to gain salvation through the care of those less fortunate than themselves; as an economic strategy, charity would calm potential social rebellion by re-distributing wealth from one class to another.[6] Of course, this system was situated on a series of gendered presumptions about care-taking, and women were charged with the unremunerated task of managing disabled lives within the confines of the household. Charity provided male members of the middle and upper classes an opportunity to use their wealth to secure divine favor in the public realms, while also keeping the poor from growing desperate and unruly. Although Winthrop phrases this social obligation as most taxing upon the wealthy, the poor become objects of beneficence managed by the rich rather than determining their own level of necessity: "Thou must observe whether thy brother hath present or probable or possible means of repaying thee, if there be none of those, thou must give him according to his necessity, rather then lend him as he requires; if he hath present means of repaying thee, thou art to look at him not as an act of mercy, but by way of Commerce, wherein thou arte to walk by the rule of justice; but if his means of repaying thee be only probable or possible, then is hee an object of thy mercy, thou must lend him, though there be danger of losing it" (1997, 38).

The practice of "charitable lending" effectively functioned as the first

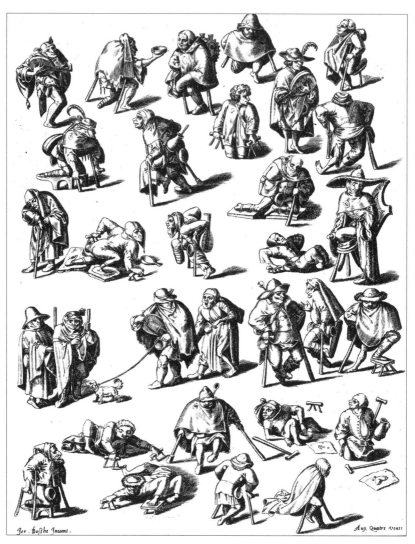

HIERONYMUS COCK, «BEGGARS STUDY» (CA. 1550), PROBABLY COPIED FROM
PIETER BRUEGHEL THE ELDER

safety net for the poor. Most important, in each case charity would serve dominant interests by placing the giver in the position of benevolent host to those struggling at the margins of subsistence. Although the United States would go on to enshrine the ideal of a "classless society" as one of its founding myths, "A Modell of Christian Charity" demonstrates that class ideologies arrived fully articulated with the earliest settlers. As lawyer turned preacher, Winthrop in his sermon likened Christian charity to a legal contract, or "binding covenant," among classes and penitents in order to assure that charity's operations would remain intact.[7] Thus, the Puritan settlement instituted a critical relationship between economic and religious orders that has remained in force to the present.

In providing a social vision that recognizes charity as a mechanism of social control, the Puritans established a founding cultural system that would cater to the needs of key social actors—namely, the wealthy who tended to become corrupt from accumulation and the attendant hoarding of social power, and the poor and "sick" who were excluded from productive labor through the combination of lack of opportunity and/or limited capacity. *Charity would provide the social salve for alleviating hardship on both ends of the economic spectrum.* In doing so, it would persist in U.S. culture as a most prized force of social mediation. Charity promised to cleanse a public space that would otherwise tend toward corruption and disquiet. It would maintain this pivotal position into the nineteenth century as the one social value on which many Americans could agree.

Yet, as economic disparities grew wider and charity registers expanded, the adequacy of public assistance began to come under attack. For instance, in 1833 John Yates, secretary of the state of New York, published a scathing report on the condition of the city's poor, whom he depicted as being ruthlessly treated by a callous economic system and further infantilized by increasing levels of public aid.[8] By the mid-nineteenth century critiques of charity became more numerous as charity's benevolent façade began to show signs of wear. Arguments over the conversion of slaves into wage laborers and the growth in alms-crying focused on what social historians have called "contract" language. In a society presumably based on the freedom to work and sell one's labor capacities, suspicions developed around the meaning of mandated labor. If one had to work in the postrevolutionary United States, then just how "voluntary" could the act of labor be? If not everyone was provided the same opportunity to labor—especially former slaves, women, and disabled people—then what distinguished postslavery America from the pre–Civil War era? If employment was a contract of exchange between capitalists and their laboring forces, then what was the place of those who were recognized as dependent on the state for their subsistence? How could charity be dispensed in a way that not provide state-sponsored subsistence as an alternative to a laboring life?

Melville's *The Confidence-Man* intervenes in a growing national debate over the inequalities of capitalism and the presumably excessive dependencies of "the needy," turning the tables on charity as an insidious social invention. Beyond the initial focus on the Deaf-Mute's admonitions on charity, there are myriad episodes of destitute begging and charity-seeking aboard the *Fidèle*: Black Guinea's pitch-penny performance; the almsgiving episode between the merchant with a traumatic brain injury and the man with the weed; the Widow and Orphan Asylum scam; the World's Charity (more on this exchange later); the man in gray's solicitation of the charitable woman in the ladies' saloon; the herb doctor's peddling of Omni-Balsamic Reinvigorator to those who might otherwise become a "burdensome care" (100); the soldier of fortune Thomas Fry's story of judicial neglect that turns him into a begging cripple on crutches; Charlemont's inexplicable descent into madness; and China Aster's tale of unforgiven debt at the hands of the shoemaker Orchis, among others. While most period critiques of charity centered on the system's encouragement of dependency on social handouts, *The Confidence-Man* exposes charity as premised on the maintenance of economic inequality. In each scene Melville moves from a request for help on behalf of those struck by "calamities against which no integrity, no forethought, no energy, no genius, no piety, could guard" (29), to the elaboration of an opportunistic deception on the part of the charitable solicitor. In this sense, the narrative continuously follows the practice of charity out into its social alter ego, the confidence game, as a foundation on which the edifice of capitalism rests.

CHARITY IN A PARASITIC ECONOMY Charity ushers in a division between hosts (those who produce and consume in equal amounts) and parasites (those who consume without replenishing what they use up). While capitalism narrates social aid recipients as parasitic upon the productive labor and tax dollars of the majority, it does so while dissimulating the dependencies of the middle and upper classes on the poor. With the development of organized charity agencies in the nineteenth century, the management of "social dependents" became legitimated as an occupation and provided stable professional careers for middle-class professionals. In doing so, the management of charity cases buoyed the economic livelihood of numerous public and private administrators who were financially dependent on the oversight of those in "need." In this sense, the distinction between host and parasite proves a fiction of exchange-based systems seeking to justify the capitalist and working classes as appropriate beneficiaries of their own productive labor capacities.

The philosopher Michel Serres describes the inequities of charity as part and parcel of an economic exchange economy whose controlling social relationship is one of hosts to parasites. Within this characterization of the

economic logic undergirding capitalism, the host is exalted as a virtuous social force at the expense of those who receive his charity: "To give without
receipt in kind is to give oneself honor and virtue, to display one's power:
that is called charity" (1982a, 6). The recipients of the host's beneficence find
themselves at a loss to reciprocate in kind for "the counterpart of charity, of
the gift without counterpart, is the whole of the poor man's conduct. This
is the only disrupting gesture where one can short-circuit the law: to give
words for goods, but the word is sacred" (1982a, 6). However, since words
are ephemeral rather than substantive (unlike the gift of food or money), the
gift of the host quickly metamorphoses within an exchange economy into a
scene of charity where one gives without receiving equivalent remuneration.

In the place of this exchange economy model, Serres proposes the paradigm of parasitic economies in which all relationships prove interdependent,
and the division between those who produce and those who consume proves
unviable.[9] As an alternative to representations of the parasite as "an abusive
guest [who] partakes of the host's meal, consumes food, and gives only words,
conversation, in return" (1982a, xxvi), a parasitic economy turns the tables on
the power inequities between benefactors and "the needy." Rather than locate the under- and unemployed as parasites on the labor of others, Serres's
definition promotes the function of the parasite as that which keeps systems
fluid and flexible. Parasites are the forces of creative possibility; like the sacred guest of Greek myth, the parasite accepts material sustenance and returns the favor with stories of adventure that enliven the world of the host.
Thus, the parasite represents a site of invention, bringing something new
into a system of meanings that would otherwise tend toward homogeneity. At
the table, the host can maintain the fiction of pure giver only as an attempt to
deny the exotic contribution of the guest's difference. Consequently, a parasitic economic model exposes the ways in which those who are marginalized
within an exchange-based economy prove necessary to the maintenance of
a dominant culture's investment in its own benefactor status. Thus, the parasite continually threatens to surface and expose this hierarchy as a social
fiction.

Serres's paradigm provides a useful theory for an analysis of charity systems that develop during the nineteenth century in the United States. Ac-
cordingly, the plot of *The Confidence-Man* depicts society aboard the steamship *Fidèle* as engaging in a series of parasitic economic relationships, in
which con artists dupe marks, shills, and each other in a frenzy of corrupt exchanges. Yet the seemingly solid distinctions between cons, marks, and shills
continually blur as all actively participate in a chain of parasitic duplicities.

Cons become marks, marks become shills, cons become shills, marks turn into cons, and so on. Thus, while the "cripple" Black Guinea declares the man with the weed as a vouchsafe to his own authenticity as a genuinely disabled beggar, the man with the weed (presumably an avatar of the confidence man) in turn becomes a target for the confidence games of the country-merchant and the Black Rapids Coal Company stockbroker. The book unseats the reader's ability to cleanly distinguish between these familiar nineteenth-century social types by undermining the strict divisions between them. No character occupies a deterministic position with respect to the economic food chain that informs human relations on the ship, and the range of avatars that the confidence man takes on during the course of the book demonstrates the degree to which economic identities are dependent on social conventions rather than on fixed capacities. The narrative plays a shell game with the location of an elusive economic host upon whom its parasitic clientele feeds. The role of host (that which exists at the origin of a food chain, upon which others feed for their survival) ultimately proves an absent center. In a profit-based economy, parasites infest every social interaction.

The Confidence-Man upsets as many stable social relations as possible to demonstrate that power is diffuse, human hierarchies performative, and interpretations fleeting and unreliable. As Susan Ryan argues, "instead of asking, as many charity writers did, for more reliable sources of information should the supplicant's body and self-presentation prove untrustworthy, Melville explores the broader implications and hazards of that unreliability as well as the moral and social instabilities of donors" (2000, 697). Like the undulating surface of the sea in *Moby-Dick*, here the more sedentary, yet still fluid, Missouri River serves to represent a placid façade that disguises the unsteady foundation of capitalism. Not that exploitation of the disempowered by the privileged proves illusory, but rather that the locations of capital exchange are infested with parasites from one end of the social order to the other. *The Confidence-Man* ultimately seeks to expose the evolution of U.S. capitalism as a false front of rhetorical justification for every social disparity. Disability proves critical to this analysis because the incapacitated body would seem to be the one reliable object where a genuinely benevolent motive might operate. Yet, as Melville demonstrates, charity mobilized by pathos or horror at the sight of incapacity (actual or feigned) fails to inaugurate a purer model of economic relations.

By disputing the fixed cultural location of disability, *The Confidence-Man* simultaneously challenges the institution of charity itself. Charity becomes a ruse by obscuring rather than exposing the truth of social injustice, as explained by the merchant: "Truth will not be comforted. Led by dear charity, lured by sweet hope, fond fancy essays this feat; but in vain; mere dreams and ideals, they explode in your hand, leaving naught but the scorching behind!" (82). Once the reliability of the act of charity is placed into question—particularly with respect to its designation as inherent tragic embodiment and nonproductivity (the disabled characters actively participate in the economic nexus of relations aboard the ship)—then systems based upon interpretations of the body become less naturalized. As the Cosmopolitan admonishes his listeners prone to judge trustworthiness on the basis of appearances: "You do not know him, or but imperfectly. His outside deceived you; at first it came near deceiving even me. . . . His outside is but put on" (187). Historically, one of the primary qualifications of charity, as Jean Starobinski has argued, has been the complete repeal of every other human right (1997, 93). The location of charity has been consciously structured in U.S. and European cultures as a site no one would willingly occupy. As Deborah Stone explains, "the workhouse was to be so unpleasant and unattractive that no one who could possibly work would choose to enter it" (1984, 39). The destitution and social stigma of poverty was not enough; charity and the almshouse as a social institution had to prove so uncomfortable that potential recipients would "choose" to reside there only as a last resort.

Debasement became an in-built feature of the charitable relationship in which the recipient degrades himself and the benefactor grows increasingly exalted. Such a formulation of the hierarchical structuring of charity came increasingly into prominence in the nineteenth century following Adam Smith's theories of the free market system, set forth in *The Theory of Moral Sentiments* (published in 1759) and *The Wealth of Nations* (published in 1776). According to Smith, an inverse relationship of power is established where the need for assistance denigrates one human actor by turning him into an object of scorn, while the provider of assistance accumulates cultural (and spiritual) capital. Charity is first predicated on the naturalized existence of social inequities, and then goes on to exact a further social toll by stigmatizing the recipient class as dependent. In this sense, charity's social significance increases in exchange-based economies because the exchange promises to "benefit" both participants in the donor relationship while actually exalting the host at the expense of the "beneficiary."

Yet charity itself operates under ideological principles that disguise this hierarchical relationship of recipient and benefactor. Its cultural narrative inverts the terms of exchange with respect to a host/parasite economic formula by promoting the parasite as the primary benefactor of charitable acts

59

and sentiments. As the transcendentalist disciple Charlie explains to his hypothetical friend Frank, played by the confidence-man, the request for assistance rents one's humanity and lowers the recipient into the depths of dependency: "Help? To say nothing to a friend, there is something wrong about the man who wants help. There is somewhere a defect, a want, a brief, a need, a crying need, somewhere about that man" (206). *The Confidence-Man* sets out to expose such a perspective as a fraud of the nineteenth-century transcendentalist ethos of rugged individualism. Both Emerson and Thoreau produced condemnatory views of charity and those in need of public assistance. For Emerson, the dependent person was guilty of failing to realize his or her calling to self-reliance, while Thoreau saw charity as debasing the philanthropist by encouraging dependency in others.[10] In both cases, charity encourages the growth of parasites on the social order and undermines the transcendentalist ideal of self-reliance for all.

Melville explicitly challenges the debilitating narrative of dependency espoused by transcendentalists and other reformers of the period. Rather than critiquing charity as promoting excessive dependency in individuals and benefactors alike, Melville situates his critique of charity at the structural level of U.S. capitalism. In other words, *The Confidence-Man* exposes charity as existing fully within the logic of an economic system that makes all economic relationships parasitic, but disguises that fact by marking only some participants as unproductive and therefore unduly dependent. Within Melville's economic analysis, charity is to be shunned not because of its promotion of excessive dependency, but rather because it encourages the wealthier classes to buy off their responsibilities to those who have been socially and economically marginalized. As one donor to the Seminole Women's and Orphans' charity magnanimously explains, "charity was in one sense not an effort, but a luxury; against too great indulgence in which his steward, a humorist, had sometimes admonished him" (48). The story also argues that the premium value of alleviating suffering, which presumably undergirds charity, supplies the narrative of capitalist exchange with a false legitimacy.

MARKETING MORAL UPLIFT AND MISERY As catalogued earlier, numerous charity causes are promoted throughout *The Confidence-Man*. Each one narrates itself as legitimate by referencing its object of intervention as synonymous with the demonstrably needy. For instance, the Seminole Women's and Orphans' fund and the World's Charity scheme both promote the legitimacy of their causes on behalf of those who are "multiply disadvantaged"; the former cause references its recipients through the marked social categories of Native American, feminine, non-Christian, and children, while the latter promotes its cause as unproductive through the more generic categories of "pauper or heathen" (39). In both cases, Melville notes the century's tendency to shift from "a Christian-based philanthropy to a bleak and professional charity based on science and statistics" (Waugh 2001, 218). Each charity effort ties a quantifiable economic incentive to a missionary purpose in which the recipients receive their benefits in exchange for conversion to a dominant religious ideology. Increasingly, nineteenth-century U.S. charity models sought to "hand out" moral uplift and middle-class values as their primary form of "aid" to social dependents.

This emphasis on moral uplift as the capital of charitable support effectively oversaw the end of "outdoor relief," whereby social dependents were supported with cash handouts at home. In its place "indoor relief" was substituted, a system in which cash supports were ended, government or community surveillance of dependents increased, and lifestyle instruction commenced. As Henri-Jacques Stiker has argued, the absence of an economic analysis of poverty even by the mid-nineteenth century gave rise to "relief" in the form of a demand for the lower classes to mimic the behaviors, sentiments, and values of the middle class (1999, 127). With morality and religious virtue identified as the necessary ingredients to resolve poverty, physical capacities became the only viable excuse for exemption from the requirement of labor for all citizens. This renewed emphasis on bodily incapacity as the primary adjudicator of membership in the "deserving poor" precipitated the rise of medical professionals, who began to apply empirical evaluations of the incapacitated body as the basis for a scientifically authorized, deserving charitable recipient.

The evidence of the ascendancy of a medical model to underwrite U.S. systems of charity in the nineteenth century surfaces in *The Confidence-Man* through the promotion of marketable products that target the body as their primary site of intervention. Prior to the discussion of the World's Charity, the gentleman with gold buttons unveils his invention of an "invalid's easy chair" recently marketed at the World's Fair in London. Once the product is introduced as a successful moneymaker for its inventor, the discussion quickly shifts from the self-interest of a marketable product to more altruistic goals referenced by the discourse of charity:

> "Is it not charity to ease human suffering? I am, and always have been, as I always will be, I trust, in the charity business, as you call it; . . . My Protean

easy-chair is a chair so all over bejointed, behinged, and bepadded, every way so elastic, springy, and docile to the airiest touch, that in some one of its endlessly-changeable accommodations of back, seat, footboard, and arms, the most rest-less body, the body most racked, nay, I had almost added the most tormented conscience must, somehow and somewhere, find rest. Believing that I owed it to suffering humanity to make known such a chair to the utmost, I scraped together my little means and off to the World's Fair with it." (38)

The design of a chair to ease the "most racked" body (and mind) places suf-fering bodies as a central premise of charity's economic authority and, in turn, as the ground on which capitalistic enterprises can stake moral claims. Commodity and therapy worlds endlessly overlap in these ways, and thus, like the "bejointed, behinged, and bepadded" easy-chair, threaten to fold into one another. Charity becomes a marketing ploy to the extent that every con game rests upon the success of the con man in marketing body com-fort, to one degree or another, as the means to alleviate social inequities. Just as the invalid's chair promises to be so "elastic, springy, and docile to the airiest touch," charity promotes its ability to alleviate a two-tiered economic relationship: not only must the disabled and discomforted be eased of their afflictions, but, more important, the benefactor must be relieved of concern over participation in an economic system based on body inequities. The con game is not so much duplicity at the expense of the wealthy as conspicuous donation for the purchase of moral appearance. Thus, the con man does not commit the crime of fraud in Melville's system; instead, he lets respon-sible citizens off the hook. He offers a rhetorical and monetary quick fix to entrenched social conflicts.

The quick fix as the primary exchange value of charity dominates the first half of the book.[11] In this scene the easy-chair inventor goes on to forward his own World's Charity scheme to his listener as an extension of his earlier work on a mass scale. As he wanders around the World's Fair with the confidence that his chair will prove a marketing success—after all, beleaguered con-sciences and bodies prove the most common product of industrial-based cap-italist systems—he becomes struck by an impulse to devise an even greater charitable effort. His epiphany centers upon the need to centralize charity under one global corporate system. Rather than dole out charity piecemeal and unmethodically, the man with gold buttons imagines the creation of a "grand benevolence tax upon all Mankind . . . a consolidation-tax of all possible benevolence taxes" (39). The collection of such a sum of charity monies in one centralized place would "warrant the dissolution of society, as that fund judiciously expended, not a pauper or heathen could remain the round world over" (39).

The elaboration of a plan to centralize charity relief ironically exposes the efforts of charity systems to sustain the purity of an economy that thrives on the maintenance of a debased lower-class labor pool: first, to end poverty with handouts rather than through addressing the systemic reasons for poverty's existence; second, by making charitable giving less onerous to the benefactor classes through the institution of a single taxation scheme on a global level that alleviates benefactors of all other social responsibilities to the "less fortunate"; and third, by maintaining the social and spiritual benefits of charitable donation that accrue to the donor classes by continuing to locate them in the illusory position of beneficent host. Rather than endorse a social system characterized by the producer/consumer binary, *The Confidence-Man* exposes the vaunted position of host as nothing more than the mark of the parasite. If production depends on the extraction of labor power from others and then turns around and sells its wares to alleviate the suffering that such labor induces in the bodies and minds of its citizens, capitalism depends on the very incapacities it produces to endlessly renew its own markets. Bodies are deemed worthy to participate in the market by virtue of their ability to perform labor, but then those very capacities are compromised by the demands of the labor process and need to be rehabilitated or supplanted by other able bodies. Disability is that which must be exempted and produced in a cycle of parasitic market dependencies while being marked as the preeminent sign of human insufficiency and disqualification from the social circuit.

Melville defines the producer class as that which is beset by the "burden" of the impoverished. Rather than ending poverty so that "not a pauper or heathen could remain the round world over," the World's Charity scheme would continue to enthrall those in the lower classes to the inequalities of a corrupt exchange economy. First, as the man in grey points out, the World's Charity scheme embodies a key flaw: it "would appear that, according to your world-wide scheme, the pauper not less than the nabob is required to contribute to the relief of pauperism, and the heathen not less than the Christian to the conversion of heathenism" (40). Thus, Melville exposes charity schemes as exacting a toll from the very classes targeted to receive relief and as founded on an imperialist project of religious universalism. Second, the World's Charity scheme also promises to alleviate the social burden of the upper classes by making charity a one-time requirement, thus freeing the benefactor class to pursue more pressing market concerns. In doing so, the

World's Charity would primarily seek to relieve the upper classes of the obligation to give to those produced as needy and dependent. *The Confidence-Man* demonstrates the absurdity of such a proposition as mistaking poverty for merely a lack of material means. Charity no longer functions as an effort to redistribute wealth, but rather as the rhetorical structure that allows the exploitative nature of capital relations to operate unchallenged.

In exposing all economic relations as parasitic, *The Confidence-Man* redistributes the idea of dependency as a culture-wide phenomenon no longer exclusive to those defined as incapacitated or excessively needy. Whether disability is performed or not proves less consequential than that those who successfully manipulate the system are those who recognize parasitism as the mediating condition of all exchange. As the misanthrope announces with respect to the impetus of human business interactions: "The pick-pocket, too, loves to have his fellow-creatures round him. Tut, man! no one goes into the crowd but for his end; and the end of too many is the same as the pick-pocket's—a purse" (137). But the exposé of parasitism in capitalism does not cast Melville as a budding Marxist seeking the overturn of a culture based upon corrupt economic practices. Instead, the work calls for the cultivation of a consistent skepticism that recognizes we are all parasites operating within an impure social system.

If charity systems cultivate a logic of parasitism that redounds to the disadvantage of those unemployed because of incapacity, inflexible work environments, social stigma, or unequal opportunity, then the task of a work of fiction is twofold: to provide a plot that can expose corruption as the foundation of unjust economic systems; and to populate the controlled setting of a story with those who are written out of the national script of participation. As disability came to be seen less as a matter of exotic monstrosity or divine punishment, these systems were increasingly replaced by investments in normalization. Charity recognized unemployment and its social shadow act of begging as the products of personal irresponsibility or misfortune. By attempting to banish people with disabilities from various social contexts, the nineteenth century sought to reestablish disability as invisible and thus unnatural. We conclude this chapter with a discussion of Melville's use of disability as a political device of characterization. As we have argued throughout, rather than consigning his disabled characters to the invisible margins of an exchange economy, Melville instead chose to write them back into the historical picture. His book forces its own universe to accommodate a social constituency believed to be better left out all together. This is the very goal of charity: to function as a payoff for those who will not be accommodated by workplaces or other public and private settings. Rather than force a revision of labor conditions or work mandates, for instance, charity buys off those who represent a source of conflict. Their absence from the social world is purchased to alleviate the need for more meaningful kinds of integration.

THE COMING OF EUGENICS The world of *The Confidence-Man* allows no easy solution in this regard. Disabled beggars who have been cast out from the economic system continue to make demands upon it. Their presence functions as a reminder and rejoinder to the insufficiencies of capitalism; their myriad differences diversify an increasingly standardized and homogeneous aesthetic desire taking root in the nineteenth century. By populating the steamship with multiple representatives of the disabled community Melville's story "renaturalizes" their existence within the artificially sterile world that the book critiques. As Rosemarie Garland Thomson (1997) has argued with respect to Melville's short story "Bartleby: A Tale of Wall Street," there is an encroaching atmosphere of eugenics in which bodies that do not fit find themselves in hostile social territory. The radicality of *The Confidence-Man* is found not in its social vision of a more inclusive society, but rather in its anticipation of new forms of social violence. As we will discuss in the next chapter, disability becomes the root cause of most forms of social deviance in the eugenics period. Melville's work recognizes that the path has been set for differences to be treated as pathologies. It functions as a warning to industrial America that its disregard for human variation—its open efforts to hide away those who fall short of an idealized national character—will prove disastrous as an economic, cultural, and aesthetic program.

For Melville there is nothing so empirical as variation itself, and in many ways *The Confidence-Man* can be interpreted as a sustained assault on the incessant American desire for the production of identity as an embodiment of narrow national ideals. Just as charity can be easily inverted into a façade for crass economics, and economics can make its appeal to potential consumers on behalf of noble charitable sentiments, Melville's narrative adheres to one predominant credo: the more contradictory and asymmetrical the representation of reality, the closer to truth one may stand. Or, as Susan Kuhlman has argued, "[Melville] is able to embody the notion that inconsistency is an important characteristic of the human personality" (1973, 114). In making his argument in favor of inconsistency, the narrator cites the "nonnormative" productions of nature as his proof that consistent characterization is nothing more than a market convention itself: "the author who draws a character, even though to common view incongruous in its parts, as the flying-squirrel, and, at different periods, as much at variance with it as the caterpillar is with the butterfly into which it changes, may yet, in so doing, be not false but faithful to the facts" (70).

From this perspective, "incongruous" portraiture provides a better map for the portrayal of human (as well as other kinds of) nature because it evades the problem of adhering to the static, idealized norms demanded by a popular culture weaned on physiognomic thinking. In approaching the social rejection of disability in this manner, Melville recognizes his primary opposition as located in the systematized order of the social that produces an illusion of fixity. Consequently, to be on the side of "life"—characterized by resistance to stasis and an allegiance to dynamic adaptation—one takes up residence with disability and other forms of embodied marginality as an affirming principle of destabilization. The allure of the normative, fostered by charity and other forms of economic standardization, must be tarnished to the point where differences are recognized as productive agents that cannot be consigned to the realm of the unnatural. Unlike the herb doctor who peddles his snake oil potion as "all natural," and thus a remedy to disability and disease as the antithesis of health—"Get nature, and you get well" (81)—*The Confidence-Man* recognizes the value of writing as that which opposes a version of nature as stasis. Disruption becomes a counterpoint to normalcy that would make over everything into a performance of stable identity.

Within such an analysis disability—or the body marked by excessive difference—becomes a more reliable signifier of the variation that characterizes humanity. Melville deploys an unusual cast of disabled characters on one stage in order to implode the ideology of identity in sameness. Disability as scapegoated difference—as that deviance which cannot be accommodated and therefore must be excluded—threatens to upset cultural investments in symmetry. As the narrator of chapter 14 argues:

> If reason be judge, no writer has produced such inconsistent characters as nature herself has. . . . As elsewhere, experience is the only guide here; but as no one man's experience can be coextensive with *what is*, it may be unwise in every case to rest upon it. When the duck-billed beaver of Australia was first brought stuffed to England, the naturalists, appealing to their classifications maintained that there was, in reality, no such creature; the bill in the specimen must needs be, in some way artificially stuck on. But let nature, to the perplexity of the naturalists, produce her duck-billed beavers as she may, lesser authors, some may hold, have no business to be perplexing readers with duck-billed characters. (70)

The Confidence-Man sets out a preponderance of "duck-billed characters," and a striking number of them are "duck-billed" by virtue of disability—so much so that the anomalous becomes the sign of the truth in variability itself. Literary anomaly, rather than the static baseline norms of empirical science or middle-class culture, governs the representational value system of life on *Fidèle*. An array of human forms, capacities, incapacities, and differences structures the social relations among Melville's cast of characters. The narrative rejects outward appearances as indicative of anything within human beings. The desire to rely on the visible resides in our wish to superficially smooth over a world overrun with upheavals and inconsistencies—a world where surprising spring snow in March contrasts with a brown farmer's face spying from a window at daybreak. Thus, the narrative continually undermines those who profess allegiance to a faith in correspondences between exteriors and interiors—and thereby exposes the falsity of the contention that "our theory teaches us to proceed by analogy from the physical to the moral" (121). Confidence in the body as a reliable signifier is the grease that allows such a principle to function without friction despite evidence to the contrary.

An adherence to the value of difference guides Melville's writings during the 1850s. As Samuel Otter explains, "[Melville] details what Foucault has called 'the nomination of the visible' . . . a world of definition, coherence, and difference [that] became located in the skin and the skull" (1999, 5). *The Confidence-Man* takes up a war with empirical norms of the body and promotes literature as producing a better empiricism of human idiosyncrasy in the realm of mimesis. The space of literature provides Melville with the flexibility to avoid slotting a dynamic humanity into fixed diagnostic categories. In a final flourish Melville uses the insufficiencies of "sciences of the surface" to provide the evidence of their own undoing:[12] "At least, something like [the value of inconsistent characterization] is claimed for certain psychological novelists; nor will the claim be here disputed. Yet, as touching this point, it may prove suggestive, that all those sallies of ingenuity, having for their end the revelation of human nature on fixed principles, have, by the best judges, been excluded with contempt from the ranks of the sciences—palmistry, physiognomy, phrenology, psychology" (71). By thwarting charity's efforts to keep disability under wraps and out of the public eye, *The Confidence-Man* creates the interference that upsets bodily appearances as a reliable medium of interpretation. In this way the tactics of Melville's writing hinge on the deformation of aesthetics as a significant register for literary innovation. As the narrator asserts in chapter 25, "the best false teeth are those made with at least two or three blemishes, the more to look like life" (140). Attention to

the existence of such blemishes recognizes disability and other socially maligned differences as occurring entirely within the register of natural human
variation. In doing so, *The Confidence-Man* exposes the social construction
of deviance as one of an array of fictions supporting charity as a restrictive
cultural locale in capitalism's repertoire of exclusionary tactics.

TWO

Subnormal Nation | The Making of a U.S. Disability Minority

'Tis a mark of God and Nature upon him, to give us warning that we should hold no Society with him, as a creature not of our original, not of our species.
A COMMENT ABOUT ALEXANDER POPE'S DISABLED BODY, QUOTED BY HIS BIOGRAPHER

The proper study of Man is man.
BRITISH PRIME MINISTER TONY BLAIR QUOTING ALEXANDER POPE AS AN ENDORSEMENT FOR THE HUMAN GENOME PROJECT

While charity sought to disguise the rampant inequities of an increasingly narrow definition of citizenship based on labor capacity, eugenics would seek a more preemptive stance toward difference. Developing as a parallel to increasingly restrictive laws and city ordinances banning vagrancy and begging, eugenics adopted a largely biological analysis of poverty and other social inequalities as a product of human deficiencies. According to early practitioners, social ills, such as unemployment, alcoholism, social unrest, prostitution, indigence, and sexual deviances, could largely be attributed to human "defects" causing the degeneration of more upstanding forms of citizenship. Such an approach cited the rampant rise of "idiocy"—a deficiency of the will, self-control, and capacity—as a scourge that needed to be handled more directly.

Eugenicists argued that ignoring the problem of "defectives in the land" (Baynton 2001) would lead to the spread of human debasement and a deterioration of the American people. This contagion-like metaphor established undesirable human variations as a symptom of wider cultural conflicts; they would be treated, for the first time in history, not in "the streets" or in almshouses where vagrancy had taken up residence, but rather in segregated training schools that were soon transformed into custodial institutions. These distinctive cultural locations for cordoning off "idiocy" from the rest of society were offshoots of asylums in that they treated human "deficiencies" as differences that could not be integrated into the flow of mainstream cultural interactions. While the first training schools for idiocy intended to offer rigorous training in personal hygiene and vocational skills, they quickly became institutions for the feebleminded as the definition of idiocy shifted from an emphasis on pathetic existence to a more menacing image. As James Trent has argued, this change in the meaning of cognitive difference was informed by deep-seated economic and social pressures that fed an increasingly medicalized approach to problems plaguing newly urbanized locales (1994, 12).

In this chapter we will explore how a tragic turn at the end of the nineteenth century led to the ascendancy of eugenics. Eugenicists effectively surrendered claims to medical objectivity in order to make judgments about the meaning and treatment of human variation. In *The Normal and the Pathological*, the medical philosopher George Canguilhem argues more generally that the medical profession in this era abandoned the project of faithfully describing the body as a neutrally adaptive organism. As a result, medical researchers capitalized on the authority to evaluate difference with reference to models of biological norms rather than as nonstigmatizing variations. Our argument does not deny the existence of physical and cognitive impairments; rather, we argue for the interpretation of differences as an expression of mutable organismic traits. As Darwin insisted in *On the Origin of Species*, variation serves the good of the species. The more variable a species is, the more flexible it is with respect to shifting environmental forces. Within this formulation, one that is central to disability studies, variations are a feature of biological elasticity rather than a discordant expression of a "natural" process gone awry.[1]

It is no coincidence that the moment of this corruption in medical methodology identified by Canguilhem coincided with the rise of the modern eugenics movement. We argue that the science of eugenics was devoted to the designation of pathology as a transmissible characteristic of human biology. Eugenicists, who were steeped in new etiologies of abnormality and whose views were supported by statistical efforts to quantify human capacities and appearances, attempted to distinguish between benign and aberrant forms of difference. Eugenics functioned as a *predictive* discourse in that its primary impetus was the anticipatory identification of aberrancies that should be eradicated from the face of the Earth (to use Elaine Scarry's [1985] phrase).[2] Here we delve into the subterranean life of eugenics as a curative or rehabilitative proposition gone awry, an ideological orientation toward bodies that transformed many human differences from adaptive organisms to generational aberrations.

Mid- to late nineteenth-century eugenics authorized, anchored, and certified what we refer to as *diagnostic regimes*. Here we coin a phrase that defines the historical transition from a "curative" promise of rehabilitation to an increasingly "custodial" proposition involving the oversight of pathologized groups viewed as nonnormative. To secure this reading, we trace one strand of U.S. disability history (the shared European and American violence undergirding eugenic practices against different bodies and minds) as precedent for each of the cultural locations of disability discussed in the chapters that follow.

INSTITUTIONAL LANDSCAPES   Let us begin with a brief look at the implementation of asylums during the early 1800s. The first U.S. state-sponsored asylums began as rehabilitative institutions for the insane. Based upon a transcendentalist belief that immersion in unspoiled Nature could cure beleaguered citizens reeling from the impact of a burgeoning industrial environment, American asylums were designed as rural sanctuaries on the outskirts of towns. Very quickly, however, asylum supervisors had to admit that this mission proved a failure: pastoral cures did not manifest the desired results, and residents often failed to return to their communities to pursue integrated lives. Nonetheless, as historian David Rothman points out, such institutions had already become fixtures in the American landscape. "The number of patients swelled and the size of the building increased. Once again an institution survived long after its original promise [of cure] had dissolved" (1971, 265).

Asylums soon became custodial rather than curative operations. Persons designated as "defective" found that a temporary stay to effect a cure invariably metamorphosed into a permanent imprisonment when their disorders refused to vanish. By the mid-nineteenth century, when the institutionalized populations had largely demonstrated their failure to become cured, psychiatrists organized themselves as professionals around a humanitarian premise

71

of scientifically supervising "defective" humanity. This effort to salvage an imprisoning regime proved ambiguous at best. As Foucault points out, the managerial assignment of "defectives" to the cognitive sciences resulted in the elaboration of a vast apparatus that translated "the sordid business of punishing into the fine profession of curing" (2003, 23). In doing so, the psychiatrist "really becomes a judge; he really undertakes an investigation, and not at the level of the individual's legal responsibility, but of his or her real guilt" (that is, a person's culpability for the possession of a discordant biology as the origin of personal and social dysfunction). Psychiatry's humanitarian rescue mission—like the original curative premises of the asylum movement it replaced—quickly devolved into a regime of intensive evaluation and internment of incarcerated bodies.

This brief overview shows that, historically, diagnostic classifications based upon pathology give way to punitive methodological strategies that subjugate the very populations they intend to rescue. Within these historical schemas what we refer to today as physical, sensory, and cognitive disability provides two paradoxical outcomes with respect to the medical orders that construct them. First, those labeled as recipients of curative interventions tend to suffer from the residual taint of their pathological identifications, but they equally fail to benefit from the initial promises of diagnostic regimes. Second, those who occupy medically based classifications of deviance serve as models for a more general understanding of human biology even as they are excluded from interaction with "healthy" citizens. The relationship between scientific diagnostic practices and pathological social consequences informs our analysis of eugenics as a predecessor practice to today's disability management and research practices.

THE ASCENDANCY OF EUGENICS   From 1890 to 1930 the U.S. intelligence quotient dropped precipitously—not, we would argue, as a result of anything inherent in the cognitive capacities of the country's populations. Rather, the drop resulted from the wide application of an extensive diagnostic regime of defective intelligence and the creation of a scientific furor around disabled people in our midst.[3] IQ testing provided the critical assessment tool that gave birth to the modern eugenics movement, for the identification of "defective persons" relied upon the establishment of a measurable baseline that separated normal from subnormal human actors. Such an ideology informs what Stephen J. Gould identifies as the critical fallacy of species differentiation via the measurement of intelligence: "no single number could possibly express general human worth, and the entire concept of IQ as a unitary biological property [is] nonsense" (Gould 1996 [1981], 22). Unlike physical characteristics, intelligence—which one of the leading eugenics practitioners, H. H. Goddard, defined as an "all-around innate mental efficiency" (1914, 557)—had not been certified as a transmissible feature of heredity. Testing, the rediscovery of Mendel's dominant/recessive gene theory, Darwin's theories of evolutionary gradualism, saltationist theories of radical organismic differentiation (facet-flipping), and the detailed chronicling of family tree data by fieldworkers placed a theory of hereditary intelligence and the potential eradication of disability within the grasp of *fin-de-siècle* U.S. and European researchers. Newly professionalized scientific disciplines, along with social work and its various therapeutic spin-offs, all flocked to participate in the identification, care, and training of those labeled "feebleminded." This frenzy of assessment produced, for a time, a "subnormal nation" out of the invention of a heretofore undesignated "defective" minority. "Defectives" threatened to undermine the country, cried eugenicists. The scientific identification of those who inhabited subnormal biologies and minds ultimately plunged the nation into a justification for institutionalizing, sterilizing, and destroying the lives of those classified as inferior humanity.

U.S. eugenics developed as a hegemonic formula from an array of Victorian ideologies. These included proliferating institutions for the incarceration of "defective" citizens; the ascendancy of neo-Darwinism (or social Darwinism) in relation to the purification of human hereditary stock; the passage of restrictive immigration laws regarding citizens with "deviant" bodies or those originating from "inferior" cultures; the dissolution of out-charity as a common cultural practice for mediating economic disparities between rich and poor; the rise of industries that promoted the concept of labor efficiency as the premium value of a contributing citizen; and the successful professionalization of U.S. medicine, psychiatry, neurology, and public health.[4]

To understand the extent to which eugenics functioned as an umbrella beneath which other pathologizing fields gathered, we must recognize that this period saw the consolidation of an ideological force of cultivated allegiances across myriad disciplines. Eugenics can be recognized as a quintessential example of hegemony. Contemporary political theorists, such as Laclau and Mouffe, formulate the Gramscian concept of hegemony as the intersection of contingent social forces that coalesce, for a time, in a unified movement of collective objectives. We will analyze eugenics as the hegemonic formation of exclusionary practices based on scientific formulas of deviancy. The movement sought to secure the professional stability of a variety

73

of disciplinary adherents at the expense of those individuals represented as functioning inadequately within a rapidly urbanizing capitalist economy. Eugenics was a veritable machine in the garden, seeking to weed out those considered unfit products of an evolutionary process.

The articulation of disabled people as a measurable expression of hereditary defect provided a rallying point for diagnostic professionals of all stripes. The newfound capacity to objectively measure intelligence handed diagnosticians a tool that all but ensured a radical increase in those identified as pathological or deviant. Identification of defect grew increasingly common, until eugenics practitioners found themselves including an ever-expanding population in the category of "feebleminded." The tools of hereditary diagnosis—field notes, IQ tests, family pedigree trees, behavioral and physical assessment, neighborhood gossip—gave eugenicists a renewed social impetus for proliferating pathological classifications upon the bodies and minds of an array of social Others: immigrants; unemployed citizens; sex industry workers; inmates of prisons, jails, asylums, and poorhouses; residents of orphanages and finishing schools, and ultimately even those who were underachieving in the public school system. The evolution of a science of heredity provided a foundation for the development of an increasingly poisoned social atmosphere with respect to the treatment of citizens with disabilities as a general descriptor for social undesirables. Yet, unlike other critical studies of this period, which regard disability as a slander upon otherwise *able* populations, our argument positions disabled people as unjustly mired within their own dehumanizing classifications. In taking this approach, we situate disability not as a marker of inferiority, but rather as representing an array of maligned differences akin to other socially denigrated communities.

DEFECTIVE SCIENCE American eugenics laid bare the social and national goals newly claimed for medical practices. It promised an empirically sound, cross-disciplinary arena for identifying "defectives" viewed as a threat to the purity of a modern nation-state. Turn-of-the-century diagnosticians came to rely on the value of bureaucratic surveillance tools, such as census data, medical catalogues, and intelligence testing. This collocation of data from the 1870s forward was accompanied by international comparisons of population trends and life and death rates, and by regulated and state-funded confinement practices. The result was a new and unwieldy set of pathological medical categories.

This growing taxonomy of pathologies consolidated physical, cognitive, and sensory disabilities in the general category of "idiocy" (by the 1880s

THE MENTAL AFFECTIONS OF CHILDREN, IDIOCY, IMBECILITY AND INSANITY

BY

WILLIAM W. IRELAND, M.D. EDIN.

H.M. Indian Army (Retired List)
Corresponding Member of the Psychiatric Society of St Petersburg
and of the New York Medico-Legal Society
Formerly Medical Superintendent of the Scottish Institution for the Education
of Imbecile Children, and Medical Officer of Miss Mary Murray's
Institution for Girls at Preston

LONDON : J. & A. CHURCHILL, 7 GREAT MARLBOROUGH STREET
PHILADELPHIA : P. BLAKISTON, SON & CO., 1012 WALNUT ST.
1898

CONTENTS

TITLE PAGE AND TABLE OF CONTENTS FROM WILLIAM IRELAND'S «MENTAL AFFECTIONS
OF CHILDREN, IDIOCY, IMBECILITY AND INSANITY» (1898), CATALOGUING
DIAGNOSES OF IDIOCY

"feeblemindedness" would replace "idiocy" as a less "objectifying" generic nomenclature). Different bodies no longer provided evidence of the breadth of God's creation, as they had done in the pre-Enlightenment period; they now signified symptoms of the same undesirable biological phenomenon—inferior intelligence and functional capacity.[5]

In other words, "idiocy" became the foundation of all human dysfunction. As the catalogue of diagnosable anomalies expanded, medical professionals simultaneously consolidated the need for their expertise in the scientific arena and worried over the ability of any one individual or field to navigate such a dizzying number of disorders. Yet, as key practitioners in the field assured their professional audiences, "our problem is a comparatively easy one, the determining of the mentality of the various persons, that is, whether normal or feeble-minded" (Goddard 1914, 30).

With respect to the ease of identification within pathological categories, early eugenic studies promoted singular mechanisms for diagnostic identification. This simplistic schema led directly to the illusion that the numbers of mental defectives were on the rise. For instance, the British physician W. W. Ireland opened his *Mental Affections of Children* with the claim that "idiots are a much more numerous class than is generally thought" (1898, 3). To support this, Ireland provided quantitative longitudinal data on the escalating numbers of idiots in European and American countries.

Ireland's tables demonstrate several foundational factors upon which eugenicists would base their claims. First was the claim that idiots and feebleminded persons defined a distinct class of people who should be distinguished from lunatics and the general asylum population. Second, his numbers point to a surprisingly high ratio of "inferior types" now residing in Western countries. The third factor was the belief that science could perform important work by using quantitative data and statistical analyses to support arguments about the demographic distribution of pathological individuals. Finally, there was a perception that membership in both categories was rising at an alarming rate. In keeping with their European counterparts, U.S. statistical researchers calculated that the numbers of feebleminded individuals increased tenfold between 1850 and 1890. Statistical data provided critical momentum for the eugenics movement, because quantitative methods gave the best demonstration that something was going terribly awry with the country's hereditary pool. Feeblemindedness was on the rise and threatening to become "the most important single group with which the state needs to concern itself" (Anderson 1919, 1).

Later studies of the group called "feebleminded" would demonstrate that

STATISTICS OF IDIOCY 9

The following shows the increase from 1850. Total number of idiots in the United States : *

1890	1880	1870	1860	1850
95,571	76,895	24,485	11,080	9149

The number of feeble-minded persons per 1,000,000 of population :

1890	1880	1870	1860	1850
1526	1533	636	602	681

In 1897 there were in twenty-four State institutions for the feeble-minded, 8492 inmates.

A COMPARATIVE CHART OF "DEFECTIVES" IN THE UNITED STATES
(FROM IRELAND 1898, 9)

the trend was continuing. For instance, in 1912 the superintendent of the Central State Hospital in Petersburg, Virginia, cited the recent census to continue arguments begun by Ireland and others: "The [U.S.] census of 1890 placed the number of feebleminded persons in the country at 95,000 and that of 1903 at about 155,000. A careful statistician has recently estimated the number at present to be about 200,000, less than 20,000 of who [sic] are cared for in special institutions. . . . Ten years ago the superintendents of American institutions for the feebleminded thought that a very conservative estimate was one to five hundred of the general population" (Drewry 1912, 3). Eugenic science quickly mastered the art of using quantitative studies to enforce an aesthetic ideology. Those who fell outside of an increasingly homogenized definition of Americanness were sequestered within the monolithic category of feeblemindedness. What studies such as these claimed to measure was a verifiable increase in idiots. What they actually measured, we will argue, was the rise of a socially constructed class of individuals who would come to be categorized as disabled. Rather than being a result of lessening biological circumstances, the sudden rise in defectives proved a product of intensifying interest in medical evaluation itself: "As our knowledge of medicine, particularly of psychiatry, and, consequently, our more accurate methods of diagnosis, has increased, a relatively larger number of persons have been found suffering from mental disease and committed to hospitals" (Drewry 1912, 9). The larger question at stake here is whether better diagnostic tools lead to identification of those who escaped classification previously, or whether diagnosis itself invents the prevalence of the object it purports to measure.

Eugenics invented a diagnostic category with extraordinarily wide parameters. Its success as a social program resulted from its ability to convince practitioners and laymen alike that the category maintained a hold in empiricism in spite of the incredible variances that it encompassed. For instance, rather than limit the classification to a finite group of abnormalities, eugenicists often quoted more general definitions of disability based on an early version of quality of life: "abnormal children [are] those afflicted with anything whatever that unfavorably affects their lives in relation to the social medium in which they live" (Drewry 1912, 22). Feeblemindedness was not only a previously unrecognized classification made operative, but also an elastic classification that encompassed many forms of "affliction."

NORMAL AND DEFECTIVE   From its roots in the study of heredity, eugenics sought to capitalize on the newfound cultural currency of medicine by tracing the origin of human defects to a shared, yet previously intangible source. "Idiocy" was identified as the elusive mouth of a biological Nile. The category promised to function as a catchall for those found to display an unacceptable degree of deviancy. In numerous eugenics publications—both popular and scientific—researchers would declare that "in a vast number of cases mental abnormalities of childhood are connected with bodily defects" (Smart 1913a, 3). While such beliefs proved common in the history of disability, in the eugenicists' arguments physical disabilities were essentially downgraded to the status of stigmata. Visible defects proved important as symptomatic pathways that led the medical practitioner more quickly than might otherwise happen to the discovery of the "feeblemindedness" residing within.

For eugenics, physical and sensory disabilities proved "merely different phases or expressions of the same fundamental inferiority" (Fernald 1912, 8). Epilepsy, deafness, blindness, paralysis, hydro- and microcephaly, trauma, tuberculosis, asthma, inflammation, sclerosis, syphilis, and cretinism all metamorphosed into the baseline expression of "mental defect" as their singular cause. Eugenics essentially tried to discount the varied expertise that would be needed to identify and treat multiple and diffuse origins of anomalies. As one of the leading practitioners counseled: "It has been suggested among psychologists that if their work is ever to mean something definite, then a certain mentality must always be called feeble-minded, and a certain other always be called normal" (State Board of Charities 1917b, 22). Devo-

tion to a singular etiology effectively grouped all forms of deviance beneath
one medicalized banner. In this manner feeblemindedness could be endlessly divided, subdivided, catalogued, and categorized, while still remaining
a catchall for abnormals. The eugenicists thus installed a binary coding system into which all human beings could be slotted: "normal" and "defective,"
or, in the reproductive sphere, those "fit" and "unfit" to breed.

The seductiveness of eugenics was embodied in the simplicity of its empirical schema. The categories of normal and defective proved enticing for
an evolving professional class who sought to lead a public campaign that
was exclusively detrimental to an entire class of disabled individuals. Eugenics promised to rid the land of all defectives by developing unbiased, empirical systems for identifying those "certain families [that] should become
extinct" (Fernald 1912, 15). The chief "accomplishment" of the eugenicists
came from their claim that defects were not singular, rarefied instances of
human anomaly, but rather the product of generations of bad breeding practices. Ritual practices of personal hygiene were translated into a social program in which the country's hereditary pool would be bathed of its impure
elements. Eugenicists argued that the cycle of hereditary transfer must be
stopped before the country could hope to get a handle on the myriad problems plaguing its shores—particularly among immigrant groups from southern and eastern Europe.

ETIOLOGY OF FEEBLEMINDEDNESS Once "idiocy" lost its scientific allure as an overarching classification, "feeblemindedness" became the
primary diagnostic category that allowed eugenics to consolidate a host of
defective types under a shared heading. Although it was articulated as a classification system for grouping individuals of inferior intellectual abilities, its
power derived from its designation of many forms of deviance as the product
of defective competence. The doctrine of eugenics consistently argued its
case on physiognomic grounds:

> The definition [of feeblemindedness], however, is incomplete unless we em-
> phasize the anatomical or physical basis of the disorder. We have to do with the
> fact of arrested or defective development of body and mind. The evidences of
> constitutional weakness, of slow growth, of inferior size, of defects in the forma-
> tion of palate, teeth, ears, skull, etc. are associated with poor sight and hearing,
> defective articulation, inability to grasp objects or to use the legs, and psychic
> weakness in any or all respects, and in many cases there is manifest disease—
> as rickets, palsy, hydrocephalus, cretinism—to which we can point as a cause.
> Imperfect as is our knowledge of the ultimate anatomical basis of these defects,

79

their general "constitutional" character is admitted, and their ultimate incurability is as distinct as is their susceptibility to amelioration. (Lincoln 1902, 2160)

We quote this passage at length to forward a disability studies–based comprehension of a phenomenon that has not yet been fully recognized in analyses of eugenics. Eugenics did not address the diagnosis of an isolated class of individuals with a purely cognitive dysfunction at base. Instead, the field promoted a slanderous ideological violence against all categories of disabled people based on stigmatized physical, sensory, and cognitive characteristics. Although in Germany eugenic ideals led to the systematic extermination of disabled people in the effort to create a purified, master race (see chapter 3), in the United States eugenicists sought rather to banish defective bodies from view and, in the process, to provide themselves with a ready-made research population. An inverse analysis was applied, by which physically disabled people presented the visible markers that presumed inferior intelligence, and those who tested positively for inferior intelligence were scrutinized—unclothed—for evidence of accompanying physical stigmata.

The physical body provided empirical evidence of an otherwise intangible disorder of the interior. "Where the germ-plasm is so acted upon as to produce mental defect we should also expect to find developmental defects of other organs of the body" (Fraser n.d., 102). An assessment of intelligence was nearly impossible without the aid of empirical measures, such as Binet's IQ tests, but visible defects could reliably indicate those who should be tested: "In the majority of cases there will be found to exist some physical abnormality, blight, or peculiarity that will give you a clue to the retarded development of the brain and mind" (Monroe 1897, 7). The reliance upon such clues was founded upon a continuing faith in the visible world that could lead one to an interpretation of an otherwise nonvisible, cognitively based capacity. All of these connections sought to emphasize that "mental subnormality is so often associated with lack of beauty, proportion, and grace in the physical body of the child, that we may say mental sub-normality and physical anomalies go hand in hand" (Farrell 1912, 14). The linkage between visible defects and subnormal intelligence proved critical to the development of eugenics methodology. Without this pairing detection was much more difficult.

Three primary classifications of defective were grouped under the heading of feeblemindedness: "the idiot, the imbecile, and the [moron]. All these represent various degrees of arrested development" (Drewry 1912, 1). Those subject to feeblemindedness were considered not merely impaired in their cognitive capacities. Their mental development was inexorably halted at a premature age: "from one aspect it seems that the condition is more as tho some poison, for instance, had suddenly been injected into the system which stopped the development of the brain uniformly throughout" (Goddard 1914, 547). The key factor in the diagnosis of feeblemindedness was arrival at a mental plateau that could not be superseded by any amount of training. Thus, the measurement of intelligence not only attempted to quantify a multi-variant phenomenon, it also imposed a deterministic boundary upon mental development itself.

Eugenicists defined each of the three categories with respect to the mean age of mental development that "afflicted" individuals attained. Overall, the feebleminded showed a degree of arrested development that placed mental intelligence at least four years behind an individual's chronological age (most argued that three years' arrested development was sufficient, but the extra year helped secure a further "conservatism" that enabled eugenicists to argue that they were pursuing a strict line of diagnosis). More specifically, "morons" were those who did not develop beyond a twelve-year-old's intellectual capacity; "imbeciles" were stuck at a mental plateau of age seven or eight; and "idiots," the most enfeebled of the group, never surpassed the mental capacity of a two-year-old. As E. A. Doll explained, subnormal intelligence followed one of two "retardation curves": "First, those who develop at a normal rate to a certain ultimate limit, mental age equaling chronological age as measured by intelligence tests, and then cease to develop or even drop back a little; and second, those who develop at a retarded rate to an ultimate limit and then cease developing" (1916b, 1).

A static principle of cognition informed eugenicist ideology. The dualistic etiology of normal and feebleminded erased a continuum of human cognitive development in favor of an inhumanly narrow, binary compartmentalization. In each case, feebleminded persons found themselves incapable of fairly competing with their fellow citizens for jobs, food, housing, and education. Morons (also referred to generically as feebleminded) were capable of being trained and even working independently, but they could never fairly compete with normal individuals (Drewry 1912, 2). Imbeciles could perform menial tasks and other "useful things" but needed to be kept under "constant supervision." Idiots proved "utterly helpless and dependent"— those who could not effectively avoid the most common dangers that beset human beings in an increasingly mechanized age.

Such classifications today resound with the unscientific cast of denigrating social epithets. However, they functioned as empirical designations of this period and help to reveal what Dorothy Nelkin explains as the buried

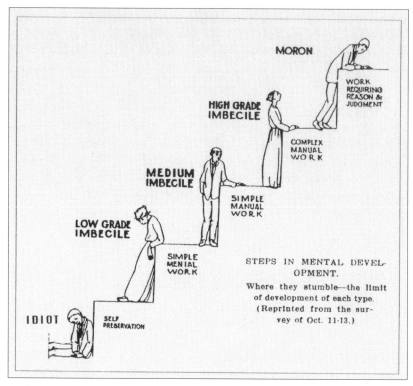

"STEPS IN MENTAL DEVELOPMENT," A DIAGRAM OF PLATEAUS OF MENTAL DEVELOPMENT
FOR EACH CATEGORY OF FEEBLEMINDEDNESS (COURTESY OF THE SMITH ELY JELLIFFE
EUGENICS COLLECTION)

implications in the "images projected by scientists in their own communications" (1995, 182). In this manner, even if we can argue that the scientific cast of such terminology is lost as they cross boundaries from research to public contexts, we are still left to contemplate the ideological assumptions invested in the scientific language games that construct disabled people. The division between biological and social discourses proves permeable because empirical characterizations must be filtered through the social consciousness of researchers and practitioners. Consequently, diagnoses inevitably originate — and are received — as imbued with value-laden characterizations.

Not only were disabled individuals endowed with a tainted heredity, but through science they were provided with labels that would undermine their individual and collective humanity even as they served as the subjects of scientific research. Researchers derided their clientele even as they wrestled to maintain a grasp on empirical objectivity: "Feeblemindedness is not an entity; it must be conceived as a disease of the deficiency group" (Stevenson 1925, 5). Likewise, Austin Freeman drew out the logical, discriminatory underpinnings of eugenicist attitudes toward their scientific wards when he wrote that the "sub-man's" difference from "the completely normal and completely fit . . . is simply a matter of deficiency. . . . They are inferior human beings, defective mentally, morally and often physically" (1923). This tension threatened to mar the integrity of the data gathered by eugenicists from the beginning of the movement. As a result, terminology shifted during the eugenics period in an effort to evade the linguistic taint of debasing language used in the development of classification categories: "Originally called idiots, they were later designated as imbeciles and still later as feeble-minded" (Goddard 1914, 3). Ultimately such efforts to sanitize the classification effort proved futile. Even the general term *feeblemindedness* failed to erase the invective that informed eugenics ideologies.

As one ascended the classification system's various levels, one fared no better. In the highest classification level, which presumably resided just below "average intelligence," eugenicists defined feeblemindedness as a veritable "synonym of human inefficiency and one of the great sources of human wretchedness and degradation" (Fernald 1912, 3). The debasing rhetoric of eugenics produced a profound intolerance in scientists and audiences alike. As one observer argued, "the majority [of feebleminded individuals] are such stunted, misshapen, hideous, specimens, that they arouse feelings of repulsion, rather than of levity" (McBroom 1923, 2). The scientific implementation of visceral language as empirical descriptors not only situated "defectives" as unacceptably deviant, it precipitated what Martin Pernick has analyzed as a medical rejection based on subjective aesthetic criteria: "while eugenics claimed to be purely objective, . . . subjective values, such as aesthetic standards of beauty and ugliness and moral attributions of responsibility, were central to eugenic constructions of hereditary disease and disability" (1996, 91). "Defectives" threatened the boundaries of acceptable deviance that the American citizen was expected to embody.

The aesthetic and subjective nature of the invention of feeblemindedness was most evident in the scientific imagination's imposition of a subjectivity upon those identified as defective. Feebleminded individuals, unlike lunatics, were not out of their senses, but they lacked sense to the degree that "comprises a group of children who are no comfort to themselves and no comfort to their parents or caretakers" (Goddard 1911, 505). This defining lack of pleasure was critical to those who diagnosed and studied the target group. To a large degree, the eugenicist campaign against defective humanity depended upon the willingness of researchers to project a state of mind for those who occupied the status of "human waste" (Anderson 1919, 9). Those characterized by a diagnosis of feeble-mindedness were essentially ventrilo-quized by eugenicists to condemn themselves. The life of a feebleminded individual was constructed as one in which "it would be better both for him and for society had he never been born" (Goddard 1914, 558).

THE "SOCIAL" MODEL OF EUGENICS   There was a social context for eugenicist arguments about the need to diagnose and exclude feeble-minded individuals in the late nineteenth and early twentieth centuries. Eu-genicists contended that traits of the feebleminded had not always invali-dated them from social, and even mainstream, participation. For instance, Goddard often repeated Binet's assertion on the relativity of human intelli-gence evaluations: "normal intelligence is a relative matter and that which is sufficient for a French peasant out in the country is not sufficient for a Frenchman in Paris" (1914, 2). In the midst of their own era's rapid industrial-ization, U.S. eugenicists took up a "progressive, modern" perspective. They premised research with advisories concerning a rapid, industrial, and even evolutionary progress of urban centers; such centers would rapidly displace "nonmodern" or "nonadaptive" humans. Eugenics argued that the country's early agrarian economy had allowed feebleminded individuals to perform the routine and relatively simple chores of the farm.[6] In addition, the dis-tance between homesteads provided a desirable buffer for hiding defectives within an isolating domestic space. In other words, an early American and predominantly rural context had effectively camouflaged feeblemindedness from social view.

With the advent of urban settings and the consolidation of greater num-bers of people in towns and cities, feeblemindedness would indicate those less capable of coping. The fast-paced lifestyles of most Americans and a less adaptable social environment effectively displaced defective individuals. As a new, manufacturing-based economy reared its head, the farm with its slower, ritualized pace of life began to vanish and with it went more flex-ible social standards, such as devotion to kin. What characterized the fee-bleminded individual, in the rhetoric of eugenics, was his or her inability to keep up with and adapt to a rapidly changing environment. Those clas-sified as feebleminded were incapable of competing on equal grounds with their normal peers. The feebleminded became synonymous with incapacity. As H. H. Goddard would reiterate throughout his voluminous body of work promoting eugenics as a moral system: "We have known that these people

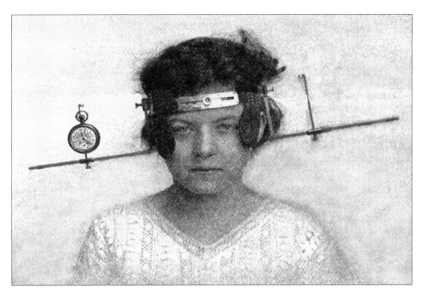

GIRL WITH AUROMETER. THE AUROMETER WAS A DEVICE TO MEASURE HEARING
LOSS, WHICH WAS THEN CORRELATED WITH DEGREE OF MENTAL IMPAIRMENT.
(FROM KNOX 1913, 1017)

did not compete successfully and that they *did not* manage their affairs with
ordinary prudence, but we have not recognized that they were fundamentally *incapable* of so doing" (1914, 5).

Thus, one could justifiably argue that changing social conditions caused
the formation of feeblemindedness as a category. Yet the diagnosis became
pivotal in a campaign waged against the displaced. Rather than target a hostile environment in the cultural locations of disability as the object of intervention, society came to use those identified within the category of feeblemindedness as the subjects upon whom the principles of eugenics were
carried out. This is one of the most disconcerting elements of eugenics as an
ideological program. While nearly all eugenicists explicitly identified the social environment as the *causal* agent of displacement, eugenicist actions continually targeted individuals rather than environments as that which needed
to be fixed. If fixing was not possible, then the affected individuals deserved
to be banished from view. Within such a schema feebleminded individuals
became social pariahs and eugenics articulated itself as a humanistic solution
to a social crisis.

The large increase in persons of "bad stock" was blamed on other causes
in addition to social environment. For example, feebleminded families were
believed to reproduce at a rate exceeding that of the normal, heterosexual,

middle-class family unit. As a forceful population management scheme, eugenics needed to generate a certain level of public paranoia in order to build support for its efforts. Eugenicists warned the public that the one "talent" bequeathed to feebleminded individuals was a prolific sexuality: "it is now an accepted fact that persons of low level mentality multiply six times faster than those on a high level" (Smart 1913a, 9). Or, as another promoter of eugenics offered, "feebleminded persons are especially prolific and reproduce their kind with greater frequency than do normal persons, and through such reproduction provide a legitimate outlet for the exercise of charitable impulses in each generation, and an endless stream of defective progeny, which are a serious drain on the resources of the nation" (Anderson 1919, 5).

Eugenics accounted for this acceleration of sexuality in part as a biological trait of feebleminded bodies. Defectives, particularly women, were the bearers of a "hyper-fertility," which made the women ideal and proficient childbearers. As Goddard pointed out, "one cannot always be sure of the chastity of these feeble-minded women" (1914, 55). Although both genders were singled out for incarceration (and, ultimately, sterilization) in institutions for the feebleminded, women became an object of eugenic scorn. "The feebleminded woman who marries is twice as prolific as the normal woman" (Fernald 1912, 7), it was claimed. Thus, defective femininity moved from a public nuisance to a bona fide threat, thereby becoming a primary target for eugenics rhetoric: "The high-grade female imbecile group is the most dangerous class. They are not capable of becoming desirable or safe members of the community. They are never able to support themselves. They are certain to become sexual offenders and to spread venereal disease or to give birth to degenerate children. Their numerous progeny usually become public charges as diseased or neglected children, imbeciles, epileptics, juvenile delinquents or later on as adult paupers or criminals" (Fernald 1912, 10). Defective women were considered unable to understand the ruses of modern masculinity and therefore more susceptible to the guile of sexual predators. Eugenicists drew up a series of equivalences for designating feebleminded women as the most dangerous of their species-type. Their uncontrolled sexuality became both the target of, and a weapon against, social efforts to curtail the ability to produce future generations of defective offspring.

Eugenicists' attitudes toward feebleminded femininity grew out of masculinist attitudes toward women's promiscuity and inherent sexual perversity in general. According to eugenicists, female feeblemindedness caused women to function at a level closer to that of instinctual animal appetites, for they pursued their sexual interests wantonly. They gravitated toward a "life of prostitution [which] is a simpler and more natural one for them. They are at the lowest ebb on the industrial market, the last hired and the first fired" (Anderson 1919, 19). According to this logic, female feeblemindedness coupled failed competitiveness with a habitual interest in sexual indiscretion. In one quantitative study of institutionalized defectives in Georgia, subnormal and feebleminded women made up 76 percent of the inmates in the State Prison Farm, 60 percent of those sent to girls' training schools, and 64 percent of those employed in brothels (Anderson 1919, 14–15, 24–25, 18–19).

If the licentiousness of feebleminded women resulted in children who became public charges as diseased, neglected, or otherwise defective progeny, or later on as adult paupers or criminals, then defective motherhood in particular and defective sexuality in general were at the root of a multitude of social problems. Eugenic researchers blamed feebleminded parents for producing a population of defective youngsters who participated in various forms of anarchy and vice. As Nancy Ordover has argued, criminal anthropologists such as G. Frank Lydston not only pathologized homosexuals in this period, but also children who had been exposed to impure heterosexual contacts: "The child of vice has within it, in many instances, the germ of vicious impulse, and no purifying influence can save it from following its own inherent inclinations. Men and women who seek, from mere satiety, variations of the normal method of sexual gratification, stamp their nervous systems with a malign influence which in the next generation may present itself as true sexual perversion. Acquired sexual perversion in one generation may be a true constitutional irradicable vice in the next, and this independently of gross physical aberrations" (quoted in Ordover 2003, 76). Although diagnoses of sexual perversion may exist "independently of gross physical aberrations," the existence of physical manifestations remained crucial to sexually based interventions. The connection between physical and behavioral defects was key to the sanctioning of "physical curatives," as the body offered better opportunities for the success of intervention strategies. Thus, as in the case of sexual deviances, a host of punitive surgeries were designed to "cure" deviants of their vices: "hysterectomy, vasectomy, castration, clitoridectomy, and blistering of the vulva, prepuce, or thighs were all prescribed by physicians in cases of perversion" (Ordover 2003, 76). Bodies became sites of invasive procedures and justified the further medicalization of human deficiencies as the locus of radical eugenic alterations of their material landscape.

In addition to sexuality, nearly any display of excessive aberrant behavior could be targeted as a cause of feeblemindedness. The spokesmen of the movement, such as H. H. Goddard, V. V. Anderson, and Walter Fernald, spearheaded a national campaign to identify all "social ills" as stemming from a singular source, defective intelligence: "Scientific researchers have demonstrated the positive and close relationship of feeblemindedness to many of society's most serious social problems, and have pointed the way to a possible solution of, or at least a scientific and intelligent approach to, the problems of crime and pauperism, juvenile vice, prostitution, venereal disease, etc." (Anderson 1919, 1). Crime, prostitution, poverty, unemployment, unsanitary conditions, nomadism, childhood abandonment, and insanity all could be traced back to mental inferiority. Anderson, for instance, notes that even institutionalization of defective children comes too late because "they have already become so-called 'criminals,' or juvenile delinquents, or prostitutes, or paupers, or vagrants, or insane persons" (Anderson 1919, 2).

Characteristic of these quantitative findings was an effort to correlate cultural wrongdoing with feeblemindedness itself. Like physical disabilities, crime and the costs of institutionalization were symptomatic expressions of feebleminded individuals' inability to conduct themselves in accordance with basic social laws. The eugenic approach to feeblemindedness soon crossed racial boundaries. In the wake of Reconstruction and with the displacements caused by the Great Migration, African Americans filled up the prisons and surpassed white inmate populations. In the 1830s and 1840s asylums and almshouses remained exclusively white and predominantly middle-class institutions, and the 1860s supplanted this population with lower class Irish immigrants. In the early twentieth century, however, exslave populations came to dominate both prison and asylum populations. Anderson reports that as of 1919 in Georgia, feeblemindedness was so prevalent among African American children that all the black schools in one southern Georgia county had been closed (1919, 31).

Ironically, the sheer prevalence of feeblemindedness in African American communities served to disqualify the population as viable candidates for eugenically based interventions. One could not effectively institutionalize an entire population, and thus, while African Americans were deemed racially "unfit," they largely escaped the devastation of eugenics-based practices. For instance, not until the late 1940s did African Americans with disabilities begin to be institutionalized along with their white counterparts. In this sense eugenic measures can be characterized as a predominantly intraracial move-

XXVI

Mental diagnoses of 120 negro school children

Normal........................	27
Subnormal...	80
Feebleminded...	13
Epileptic......	0
Psychopathic...	0
Total..	120

"MENTAL DIAGNOSES OF 120 NEGRO SCHOOL CHILDREN," A TABLE CLASSIFYING
AFRICAN AMERICAN "DEFECTIVES" IN ONE GEORGIA COUNTY
(FROM ANDERSON 1919, 31)

ment. Eugenics was a form of social prophylactic against members who were imagined to endanger the racial stock from the "inside." As public health historian Paul Weindling expresses it, eugenics essentially transformed the "professional sector of the middle class with the growth of responsibilities of doctors, welfare workers and psychologists" through the proliferation of "general biological values" toward their fellow citizens (1989, 6). To accomplish this goal, eugenicists consistently characterized institutions as humane solutions to the threat that people of inferior stock posed to the nation's germ plasm.

This effort to characterize institutional programs in benign terms proved in keeping with the liberal rhetoric of eugenic promoters. In order to position institutions as a desirable alternative, eugenicists often contrasted them to punitive institutions. Goddard and others argued that it was cruel to imprison individuals who were not responsible for their actions by placing them in reformatories, jails, and prisons: "We must measure intelligence. Knowing the grade of intelligence we may know the degree of responsibility. Knowing the degree of responsibility we know how to treat. . . . [P]robably 25% to 50% of the people in our prisons are mentally defective and incapable of managing their affairs with ordinary prudence" (Goddard 1914, 3, 7). Instead of imprisonment, they proposed a form of incarceration deemed more appropriate for a biologically based deviance that could not be cured, one that was supervised and managed by middle-class professionals as part of a proliferating medical industry that had infiltrated into most cultural arenas of influence.

The flourishing of institutions for the feebleminded in the first half of the twentieth century demonstrates the success of eugenicist programs. Already by 1914 thirty-six states had institutions for the feebleminded (Smith, Wilkinson, and Wagoner 1914, 36–81). Soon nearly every state could boast at least one or two structures that housed and managed their subnormal populations (Amici Curiae 2000, 4). The initial argument undergirding the construction of this new institutional formation was a proposition that "it is possible to colonize all of our feeble-minded persons under conditions in which they would be perfectly happy" (Goddard 1911, 265). Later this contention was slightly revised by more economically conscious proponents of institutionalization: "The feebleminded can be economically housed if we discard the mistaken idea of elaborate buildings and equipment. At the same time, they can be happy, useful, and contented" (Anderson 1919, 36). These exclusion-based "solutions" to human differences show the eugenicists' readiness to posit their subjects' mindset. If one could convincingly argue that those labeled feebleminded would respond enthusiastically to their impending incarceration, then the violence of the deed and the inmates' loss of liberties could be more easily sanctioned. Because their own subjectivities had already been evacuated of emotional and cognitive complexity, others could readily supply the reactions of feebleminded individuals to even the most radical forms of exclusion.

Perhaps most disconcerting about the social underpinnings of the designation of feeblemindedness was the escalating rates of incarceration of people with disabilities. By 1923 institutions for the feebleminded reported incarcerating more than 60 percent of the eighty thousand individuals who had been formally diagnosed in the category; by 1939, they reported that 74 percent were incarcerated. Like asylums in the first half of the nineteenth century, institutions for the feebleminded rapidly became fixtures in the American landscape. And again like the asylums in the 1830s with their failed cure missions, institutions for the feebleminded were founded upon an illusory notion of rehabilitation and return of improved defectives to the community. As Boston physician David Lincoln explains: "The idea, now so prevalent, that provision must be made for the custody and care of large numbers of the feebleminded, did not begin to seem important until a number of years later; not, in fact, until years of patient effort had demonstrated . . . how imperfect the results of the best training must be" (1902, 2159). This realization occurred slowly but absolutely according to eugenicist materials. In spite of its best efforts, eugenic science was forced to admit "with subject after subject, . . . that it has no future for the child or that it was suited only to select high-grade cases. We are impelled by necessity as well as by inclination to tell the truth, even if it should involve confession of failure. . . .

Interested, as we are, to the utmost in the future of the work with defectives, we would far rather say this ourselves than have the admission forced upon us by unfriendly critics" (Monroe 1897, 16). As a result, institutions for the feebleminded as a cultural location of disability transformed themselves from curative to custodial operations by the late 1890s. They thus fulfill our earlier definition of a diagnostic regime.

Institutional practices explicitly sought to extract defective citizens from participation in the social mainstream. In this regard, institutions for the feebleminded accomplished three distinct objectives: First, in conjunction with the passage of marriage and state sterilization laws, eugenics institutions participated in erasing disabled citizens from public view with the full sanction of state and federal governments. Second, through the incarceration of disabled citizens, they further reified stigmatizing beliefs about disability by preventing public intimacy with differences that might mitigate their construction as alien. Third, they posed as safe, humane places for the "treatment" of disabilities while operating essentially as research warehouses.

There is ample evidence that institutionalization proved stifling, even deadly. For example, within two months of admission more than 10 percent of those institutionalized died (Harley 1916, 3). Nonetheless, institutions for the feebleminded continued to proliferate and function as the social "cure" for "defectives in our midst." Disability proved so unwelcome that it began to operate under the conditions of a wider cultural repression. To shut away difference from public view resulted in a false assurance that disability made no claim upon public institutions regarding the complexities of access or integration. In addition, the physical removal of people with disabilities relieved the wider culture of reckoning with the nature of human variation across communities. Institutions for the feebleminded promised to restore a desired social balance to the country, while also eliminating longstanding social problems. To accomplish these ambitious goals required the cooperation of an extensive bureaucratic surveillance network that could effectively screen, evaluate, and identify citizens who threatened the progressive formula of national purity. Public schools played a central role in the identification of those who resided among the members of the subnormal nation.

EDUCATIONAL SURVEILLANCE NETWORKS Perhaps the most "successful" application of eugenicist doctrines was the establishment of an elaborate bureaucratic surveillance operation. This effort began to take shape in the late 1800s as eugenics was gaining authority as an empirical diagnostic practice. Because the field promoted the utility of its applications as a mechanism for "weeding out" previously undetectable defectives in the general population, it relied upon the oversight of public agencies to identify potential specimens for testing and segregation. Implementing such a vast social project required the involvement of public institutions with sweeping access to large numbers of American citizens—particularly children. It was Goddard who identified public schools as the natural place to conduct eugenics-based oversight, as a new cultural location of disability. At this time he was promoting the establishment of a national records office that would help employers identify potentially unproductive applicants, an effort that led to the establishment of the National Eugenics Office in Cold Spring Harbor, New York. "Our first problem then," he said, "is to recognize the moron. By suitable mental examination they must be discovered, and discovered as early as possible. This is best done by the public schools. If a child is backward he must be carefully watched" (Goddard 1914, 585).

To "carefully watch" potential and existing eugenic subjects provides an opportunity for the identification of aberrancy to metamorphose into a diagnostic regime of surveillance. Once the elaborate diagnostic mechanisms of eugenic science were in place, its practices could be extended across an array of state and federal institutions. The blurring of boundaries between medical and administrative gazes gave way to the implementation of an ideological vision with enormous social potential as a mechanism of population control. No longer an exclusive province of medical or institutional science, eugenic practices infected the governmental and pedagogical domains of public discourse. The administration and further consolidation of power largely paralleled the adoption by state and federal programs of the surveillance principles propounded by medical science.

The identification of public schools came about fairly late in the development of eugenic principles. In the United States, as well as in France and Britain, the nineteenth century oversaw the provision of the first institutions and "training schools" for feebleminded individuals, but they largely functioned as voluntary institutions for those surrendered by parents, orphanages, and almshouses as "defective" or "incorrigible." For instance, Samuel Howe established the first institution for the feebleminded in South Boston following an 1848 report on the condition of the mentally defective who did not qualify for incarceration in insane asylums. By 1894 the first school for feebleminded individuals was established in Providence, Rhode Island (Lincoln 1902, 2192). The move from institution to training school allowed for a liberal discourse to control the public perception of avowed segregation by emphasizing a move from sedentary imprisonment to educable environment. The permanent custodianship of institutionalized residents remained an avowed goal, but the function of the institutions could be narrated as less punitive, and thus, more humane.

In this sense, the nearly fifty years that saw the establishment of institutions and training schools also saw a shift in ideological approach. All operations increasingly came to believe in the value of manual exertion for residents. "Training" in these settings focused on vigorous physical and concentration exercises based upon the scheme elaborated by the French educator Séguin, who held that "sluggish intellectual functions could be aroused by energetic oft-repeated stimuli to the brain through all sensory pathways and by calisthenics to correct deformities and improve the health, posture and movements" (Cobb 1925, 1). Physically able defectives found themselves engaged in exercises of regulated marching, nature walks, weight training, gymnastics, and competitive outdoor sports. This emphasis on orderly participation during tasks of physical exertion had ameliorative effects upon incarcerated residents. What Foucault might refer to as the governmentality of the self was asserted as the explicit objective of eugenic-based institutions (2003, 48). Its achievement entailed an overall internalization of docility with each institutional resident: self-mastery over bodily functions; opportunities to exhaust an overabundance of restlessness and misplaced energy; and occupation with skills that displaced a tendency toward "sedentariness," "liability to consumption," and "undesirable sexual interests" (Lincoln 1902, 2167–69).

The use of exercise regimes as a tool for disciplining subjects also corresponds to Foucault's analysis in *The Care of the Self* with respect to personal discipline: "[a good physical regimen] . . . does not require that one institute a struggle of the soul against the body, nor even that one establish means by which the soul might defend itself from the body. Rather, it is a matter of the soul's correcting itself in order to be able to guide the body according to a law which is that of the body itself" (1988a, 140). Filling up the days of institutionalized residents with repetitive activities of physical exertion tended to produce docile defectives. Such regimens also assisted the institutions in achieving the ultimate goal of making their charges "useful" through participation in low-wage labor activities that could generate and sustain profits for institutions. Many institutions established workhouses on the premises. Numerous institutions and training schools also included colonies that set residents to work in the community.

Particularly within the U.S. context, this regimen of physical exertion came to dominate the tasks assigned to defective citizens; about three-

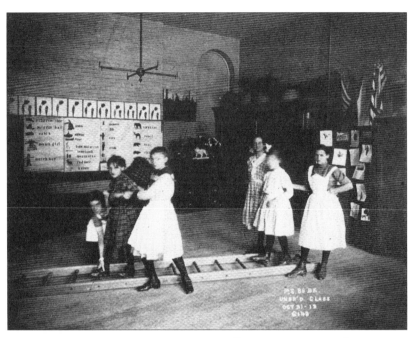

GAIT TRAINING SESSION, PART OF A PROGRAM OF "CORRECTIVE GYMNASTICS" AT THE
NEW YORK SCHOOL FOR THE FEEBLEMINDED, C. 1912 (FROM «FOURTEENTH
ANNUAL REPORT, DEPT. OF EDUCATION, CITY OF NEW YORK,
CITY SUPERINTENDENT OF SCHOOLS,» 1911–12, 16)

quarters of each school day was devoted to the improvement of motor control
and practices of personal hygiene.

> From two years of age, the defective or idiotic child may be taught with pains-
> taking care to do what other children learn by observation and imitation. The
> process of education is in most cases pursued with the following distinct pur-
> poses in view:
> 1. To develop the attention and sharpen the five senses.
> 2. To develop coordinated movements and strengthen the muscles—(a) To
> teach to walk; (b) to teach use of the hands.
> 3. To inculcate habits of cleanliness in person and dress.
> 4. To teach the patient the use of language.
> 5. To arouse the intellect by including ideas of length, weight, surface, solids,
> form, and number.
> 6. Finally, to carry the education higher, by means of studies in natural his-
> tory and all sorts of manual and industrial and moral training. (Peterson 1898,
> 682)

This general pedagogical scheme for defective children constituted the educational objectives of all institutions and training schools. The hierarchical scale of activities moves from an individualized regimen of personal upkeep to an orderly preparation of the self for the social order writ large. In other words, training of the feebleminded was predicated upon a parallel between the micro-politics of the self and the macro-politics of the social body. Although institutionalized individuals were not allowed to return to mainstream society, the society of the institution became an allegory for the larger culture. Good inmates made good citizens, even if their extraction from the social circuit was absolute and perdurable. Ironically, the overriding defect of limited intelligence was viewed as a benefit to the project of creating the ideal national subject.

UNGRADED CLASSES Eugenics sought a policing function that used the diagnostic category of defective as its weapon to enforce an inflexible normative model upon those who appeared and/or behaved demonstrably different from the majority. U.S. public schools first participated in eugenics by accepting the role of designating students who had trouble keeping up with classmates. Mandatory attendance provided schools with an unprecedented opportunity to function as an important cog in the eugenic machinery of social filtration. The classroom merged medical and educational jurisdictions in a unique formula of disciplinary convergence: "The treatment of idiots involves the employment of both physician and teacher. The adjective medico-pedagogic is made use of to designate this combination of medical and educational features for the care of defective classes" (Peterson 1898, 681). Teachers and school administrators participated as co-conspirators in the identification of potential inferiors presumably trying to pass for normal in the general classroom environment.

The simplicity of diagnostic prognosis that undergirded eugenicist ideology provided the impetus for the wide application of stigmatizing diagnostic practices. The pollution of educational methods with the authority of medical classification techniques turned classrooms into toxic atmospheres. In an 1897 report Will S. Monroe, an instructor in pedagogy and psychology in the State Normal School in Westfield, Massachusetts, sent a letter to public school teachers asking them to "observe the physical and mental defects of the children under their charge" (7). Citing another medical expert, Monroe pointed out to teachers that they should focus upon the "more noticeable characteristics of the truly feeble-minded child" as a sign of inferiority (ibid.). Teachers identified slow students, administrators passed on

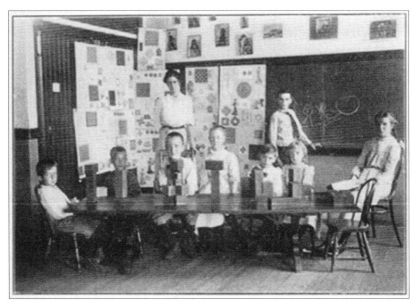

A "FEEBLEMINDED" KINDERGARTEN CLASS (COURTESY OF THE SMITH ELY JELLIFFE
EUGENICS COLLECTION)

lists of potentially feebleminded participants to eugenic authorities, and eugenic researchers implemented IQ testing to confirm the identification of "affected" individuals. Once identified, feebleminded students were placed in ungraded classes that adopted the physical training protocols developed in eugenic training schools. As the predecessor of today's special education classrooms, ungraded classes initially served as holding tanks for defective students awaiting processing into institutions for the feebleminded: "The special class should be a sieve through which those who will not be self-supporting, those who will not be law-abiding, and those who will not have proper supervision shall not pass unless to enter a custodial institution. Provision should be made to study these children and to secure their admission to an institution for defectives before they leave school to go to work" (F. Smith 1917, 73).

The first ungraded classes, established in New York City and Chicago, were intended not to provide a prolonged curriculum, but rather to segregate defectives from the mainstream school population. Such a tactic proved desirable, according to eugenicists and school administrators alike, because it relieved a burden upon both teachers and students seeking a normal educational model: "there remains as justification for the special class the advantage that appeals so much to the school superintendent—it removes the grit from the educational machine, and allows the wheels to run smoothly" (Nash and Porteus 1919, 2). Feebleminded students were believed not only to slow down the natural pace of study, but also to lower the intellectual level at which the entire class could participate. Finally, defectives required more attention from the "ordinary" teacher "who gives perhaps thirty per cent of her energy to the few feebleminded pupils she may have," so that the education of normal students was "retarded" (Fitts 1916, 1). Segregating those diagnosed as feebleminded into ungraded classrooms saved defectives from the humiliation of falling short of normalized educational expectations that the regular classroom had adopted.

Eventually, the establishment of ungraded classrooms became an institutional fixture within the public school system. Proponents of special education would ultimately argue that establishing and maintaining a separate curriculum within the public schools would prove more economically feasible than institutionalization, because students of inferior intellect could effectively be segregated within schools while continuing to live at home. In this way the U.S. model of ungraded classes in regular schools would significantly diverge from the separate educational structures of European practitioners. Advocates of ungraded classes argued against the construction of separate facilities for defective students: "The special class rather than the special school seems to meet American conditions best" (Farrell 1912, 14). Writing in 1912 the New York superintendent of ungraded classes, Elizabeth Farrell, explicated the available models of educational facilities for feebleminded children. In England, she noted, the special school is strategically isolated to prevent the "association in school of the mentally defective and the so-called normal child": "For this special school building there are separate entrances, separate playgrounds, separate gymnasiums, lavatories, passages and offices" (1912, 13). Ungraded classes, in contrast, would take place either in a more remote location within the school proper or in temporary facilities located on the school grounds. Advocates of ungraded classes partly reversed previous notions of absolute segregation by arguing that some contact between normal and feebleminded students was desirable because it would foster a sense of genuine superiority in the general student population: "May this class not be made an opportunity for the normal child to feel the obligation of the strong to the weak[?]" (Farrell 1912, 15). In addition, these interactions might contribute to a sense of charity and responsibility among those who were more fortunate.

The upshot of these discussions was not a lessening of tension around social questions concerning the handling of citizens with disabilities. Instead, discussions of identification, diagnosis, institutionalization, and absolute or partial segregation resulted in an exacerbation of restrictive measures across the country. In *Eugenical Sterilization* Harry H. Laughlin (1922), the future assistant director of the Eugenics Record Office, noted that by 1914 forty states had adopted laws prohibiting the marriage of cognitively disabled people; by 1922 fifteen states had passed compulsory sterilization laws aimed at ending the ability of physically and cognitively disabled people to reproduce; and twenty other states had considered passing eugenic sterilization laws (most received the governor's veto). Nearly twice as many women were sterilized as men. By 1963 more than sixty-three thousand individuals had been forcibly sterilized in state institutions (Amici Curiae 2000, 6). The legacy of eugenics was sweeping, systematic, and violently pathologizing because it founded its interventions on the mistaken faith in the ability to eradicate what it believed to be undesirable degrees of physical and cognitive differences from the biological record.

THE EVOLUTION OF EUGENICS   Eugenics accelerated the now common practice of using disabled people as the foundation of knowledge about biology in general, while excluding them from social belonging. The epigraphs to this chapter embody this paradox. While a famous line from the multiply disabled poet Alexander Pope can be championed as an endorsement for the curative programs of the Human Genome Project today, he was derided in his own time for his physical differences. People with disabilities, having first been diagnosed as anomalous expressions of hereditary discordance, suffer the disastrous social consequences of such attributions. Like Pope's contemporary detractors, eugenicists also argued that we should hold no society with the disabled, for they are creatures not of our original, not of our species. Disabilities provide the basis for the designation of species-typical characteristics even as they are identified as most atypical. The disabled Other is always within and without.

Such is the nature of the creation of a distinctive social minority. The social markers that constitute difference select a population for differentiation and paternalistic practices of protectionism. Yet this enfeebling discourse ultimately becomes the basis for legalized segregation. Thus, what begins in a chivalric narrative of delivery from inferiority ends in pathologization. Our goal is to use a notorious historical example to suggest a content that must not be ignored or buried as an error of the past. If eugenics galvanized its critical scientific materials during the first decade of the twentieth century, much of its momentum was borrowed from late Victorian beliefs in the science of evolution and theories about the hereditary passage of inferior intelligence as a quantifiable entity. "The term *genetics* was coined in 1905 and *gene* in 1909. In 1915 T. H. Morgan published *The Mechanics of Mendelian Heredity*; in 1916 the first genetics journal was founded" (Fox-Keller 1996, 4). Eugenicists boasted about the establishment of courses and degrees in eugenics and genetics offered by some of the country's most prestigious schools: Columbia, Harvard, Princeton, Brown, University of Chicago, University of Illinois at Urbana, and University of California, Berkeley (Laughlin 1922, 393). This conjoined birth was not coincidental; nor were the two discourses radically distinct from each other; both took as their primary object of study the "problem" of hereditary transmission. Diagnostic regimes have historically led to more stigmatization once the curative promise has been abandoned. Our ability to erase organically embedded characteristics that are integral to the functioning of bodies and minds ultimately threatens the very core of our viability as biologically based beings in the first place.

THREE

The Eugenic Atlantic | Disability and the Making of an International Science

In recent decades a significant body of historical research has been produced on the devastation of ethnic and sexual minority communities during the Nazi regime, such as Jewish, Romany, and gay peoples. Holocaust scholars have probed the intricacies of the psychological, social, political/economic, and ideological contours of Germany in the 1930s and 1940s. This body of scholarship has proven critical to a sobering contemplation of Western violence against social Others. The Holocaust, according to Saul Friedlander, has become a touchstone for theorizing the violent underpinnings of twentieth-century racist mindsets: "It could be that in our century of genocide and mass criminality, apart from its specific historical context, the extermination of the Jews of Europe is perceived by many as the ultimate standard of evil, against which all degrees of evil may be measured" (1997, 1).

Yet Holocaust studies has only recently begun to look at the systematic slaughter of disabled people under the Nazi regime. A study of disability should play a critical role in any effort to comprehend the nature and mechanisms of the Nazi Holocaust. In our view eugenics, as the science of racial purification and the elimination of human "defects," is pivotal to apprehending this deadly period in a collective Western history. Eugenics became the site where beliefs about racial and biological inferiority dovetailed for a period of approximately one hundred fifty years in the cultural location that Paul Gilroy (1995) has named the "Black Atlantic."

In this chapter we fold the cultural location of disability into this cross-national equation. Although discriminatory practices against racial populations are not identical with those enacted on disabled people within the eugenics period, eugenic ideology nonetheless exhibited racist components, and racist ideologies can tell us something about the cultural construction of disability. By the end of the eighteenth century racial and disability ideologies buttressed beliefs about the inferiority of both populations. By drawing upon Gilroy's emphasis on transatlantic traffic in racial thinking as a site to include comparative discussions of disabled peoples, we offer some parallels between race and disability as dehumanizing formations. In identifying a "Eugenic Atlantic," we also refer to Gilroy's analysis of cultural crossings in order to recognize the social construction of marginalized populations designated by virtue of their presumed biologically based inferiorities. Our analysis of a "Eugenic Atlantic" seeks to fold disability and race into a mutual project of human exclusion based upon scientific management systems successively developed within modernity. From the end of the eighteenth century to the conclusion of World War II, bodies designated as defective became the focal point of European and American efforts to engineer a "healthy" body politic. While fears of racial, sexual, and gendered "weakness" served as the spokes of this belief system, disability, as a synonym for biological (or in-built) inferiority, functioned as the hub that provided cross-cultural utility.

EUGENICS ERASURE To a significant extent the failure to locate the origins of the Holocaust with the murder of disabled people stems from a lack of serious engagement with the hegemony of eugenic science and thinking in the West. Scholars persist in casting eugenics as "quack science" (Gould 1996 [1981]) or a "bad idea" (E. Carlson 2001), thus permitting it to pass as a historical aberration. Some excellent studies have been published on the eugenics movement in specific countries, among them Paul Weindling's *Health, Race and German Politics between National Unification and Nazism, 1870–1945* (1989), Richard Soloway's *Demography and Degeneration: Eugenics and the Declining Birthrate in Twentieth-Century Britain* (1990), James Trent's *Inventing the Feeble Mind: A History of Mental Retar-*

dation in the United States (1994), Diane Paul's *Controlling Human Heredity: 1856 to the Present* (1995), Daniel Kevles's *In the Name of Eugenics* (1995), Martin Pernick's *Black Stork: Eugenics and the Death of "Defective" Babies in American Medicine and Motion Pictures since 1915* (1996), Anne Kerr and Tom Shakespeare's *Genetic Politics: From Eugenics to Genome* (2002), Nancy Ordover's *American Eugenics: Race, Queer Anatomy, and the Science of Nationalism* (2003), Edwin Black's *War against the Weak: Eugenics and America's Campaign to Create a Master Race* (2003). Still, eugenics has failed to attain a substantive place in the contemporary comparative history of science. Few college or secondary school classes take up eugenics in a meaningful way (if at all). Thus, one principal barometer in the contemporary history of disabled people has been erased, ignored, or, even worse, diminished.[1]

In many ways this erasure is a symptom of the failure of Western educational systems to engage in a thoroughgoing analysis of beliefs about disability. It results in the abandonment of disability to the deficit models that abound in the pivotal locations of medical and rehabilitation sciences—as well as in the perpetuation of deficit measures developed within, and as substantial "proofs" for, eugenic science. Our cultural ambivalence about the status of disabled people bolsters a desire to ignore the disastrous legacies evident in a history of collecting, defining, naming, measuring, and managing them as "feebleminded," "subnormal," or simply "defective" humanity.

We see this larger disciplinary and pedagogical disregard for the eugenics movement as involving three distinct, though related, factors. The first is the persistent ambivalence in Europe and North America about the value of disabled lives. When the Nuremberg trials effectively ruled out the prosecution of those who participated in the Nazi euthanasia program from its legal jurisdiction (Lifton 2000, 18; Weindling 1989, 565), the decision solidified, rather than interrogated, a key element of Nazi ideology: namely, that the extermination of disabled people in Germany and the occupied countries was unconnected to the horror of the concentration camps. As Weindling (1989) points out, "although there was horror at Nazi atrocities, most academic and professional institutions survived unscathed, or were reconstituted in such a way that social interests were left intact. . . . There were remarkable continuities in the personnel and administrative structures of public health services and many leading racial hygenists were reinstated between 1946 and the early 1950s as 'human geneticists'" (565–66). In other words, one could effectively assume that if the Nazis had not moved from the persecution of biological and cognitive "deviants" to the extermination of racial, ethnic, and sexual minorities, the imaginary line between "medical intervention" and murder would not have been crossed (see our film *A World without Bodies* [2002] for a further iteration of this argument). Thus, the need for war crimes trials might have been rendered moot.

Second, the eugenics movement was a truly transatlantic affair. As Gilroy contends in *Against Race*, even the most liberal and leftist histories have reproduced the nation-state as an absolute boundary in the modern analysis of socially hybrid multinational identities (2001, 64–65). With this in mind, we argue that an adequate account of the modern history of disabled people has failed to materialize because disability occupies a dual status as the most insular and also the most transcultural of phenomena. While all modern nation-states have mulled over the appropriate fate of their disabled populations within the cultural locations of stringent national borders, disability served the space of the Eugenic Atlantic as a primary catalyst for international collaboration. In this way, the science and social policy of disability became part and parcel of what Daniel T. Rodgers (1998) has called "Atlantic crossings": "a distinctive era in the American past, in which American social politics were tied to social political debates and endeavors in Europe through a web of rivalry and exchange" (5). Thus, the cultural location of disability during the eugenics period was imported and exported across European and American nations, making its analysis more elusive through its political and scientific ubiquity.

Lest the term *collaboration* be misunderstood here, we intend it to suggest an unprecedented level of scientific and governmental exchange over what to do with those designated with physical, sensory, and cognitive "defects." In other words, international discussions of disabled people, particularly during the first half of the twentieth century, provided important opportunities for cross-cultural exchange, but largely at the expense of disabled people themselves. Eugenics, primarily articulated as a benign practice to "help" take care of disabled people who were by definition incapable of caring for themselves, provided a fertile field for multinational cooperative engagement at the ideological level of biological aesthetics. By adopting a catalogue of "defective" conditions—epilepsy, feeblemindedness, deafness, blindness, congenital impairment, chronic depression, schizophrenia, alcoholism—European and North American eugenics engaged in a shared campaign of biological targeting that addressed deviance as a scourge to be banished from a transatlantic hereditary pool. *Such a multinational conversation demonstrates that while disabled people were effectively immobilized from participating in inter- and intra-country movements, the discourse of disability functioned in a diasporic manner.* Participating countries were responsible for overseeing the management of their own aberrant citizens, but the transnational nature of the phenomenon allowed European and North American nations to point to each other as a justification for increasingly restrictive, and ultimately pathological, measures.

Third, with the exception of the work on Nazi eugenics by historians such as Michael Burleigh (1994), Henry Friedlander (1997), Hugh Gallagher (1989), Robert Lifton (2000), Robert Proctor (1988), and Paul Weindling (1989), there has been a lack of historical scholarship in English on the treatment of disabled people in the period leading up to and during the Holocaust. The scholarly encounter with the devastation of people with disabilities in World War II has surfaced largely as a result of interest in the workings of Nazi medicine as the most egregious violation of the Hippocratic oath's injunction to "first, do no harm"—that which German historian Benno Mueller-Hill has termed "murderous science" (1988). This approach has yielded important insights into a medical mindset of the period that developed in Germany, while largely overlooking the ideological seeds of this perspective in other European and North American countries. Like eugenics before it, Nazi medicine has been chronicled as an unprecedented aberration of the healing professions—particularly when we include the collaboration of nursing (McFarland-Icke 1999), psychiatry (Lapon 1986), social work, and the therapeutic sciences (Lifton 2000) in the killing practices.

We do not wish to challenge such a claim because it turns pathology away from disabled bodies and places it where it rightly belongs within the health professions of the period. Nonetheless, the historical re-creation of these horrific events has engendered its own problems. First, the contours of this shared narrative by historians allows Germany to be effectively sealed off from its participation in international scientific premises about bodies. Participation in the Eugenic Atlantic contaminated the shared cultural location of disability and turned disabled persons into pariahs at the population level. Even among countries that were engaged military enemies at the time, scientific and cultural agreement about the menace of "defectives" transcended battlefields and diplomatic impasses as an ideological formation. Second, one senses a discomforting ambivalence in a majority of these studies with respect to the disabled "victims" who were subject to them. The general tone that pervades contemporary euthanasia studies, as Henry Friedlander contends, is one in which "handicapped" people "were not mentally deficient but only suffered from a physical deformity; their disfigurement condemned them" (1997, 170). The characterization positions people with cognitive disabilities at the farthest degree of subnormalcy while also portraying physically disabled people as suffering victims of their own conditions. To highlight the devastation wrought by Nazi medicine, contemporary historians, with little direct knowledge of disabled persons or disability studies, have disturbingly echoed euthanasia movements in their characterization of people with disabilities as pathetic victims of a murderous regime *and* of their own tragic embodiment.

Friedlander, one of the most progressive of the Holocaust historians in this area, argues that "the Nazis' victims did not suffer from diseases that were terminal or from disabilities that were necessarily incurable" (1997, xxi). This is a repeated contention in current Holocaust scholarship that tries to establish the possibility of a successful remediation of disability as evidence that those killed were not eternally outside the eugenics domain of normalization. But disability studies must contest even this assumption as part of a scholarship that accepts normalization as the adjudicator of human value. One must ask if murder would be acceptable (or, at least, less egregious) if those exterminated had terminal illnesses or nonremediable disabilities. The phrasing implies that such situations would complicate our ability to condemn these actions fully.

Nevertheless, the scholarship on this formerly buried area of history provides important materials for re-creating another key aspect of disability history. This overdue attention to disability issues has been in large part the result of work by international and German disability studies scholars who have addressed assumptions within medical models leading to stigmatizing attitudes, yes, but also to disability genocide. In addition, there is considerable German research on the Nazi euthanasia campaign, which has yet to be translated into English. Thus, critical work by scholars such as Ernst Klee, Gotz Aly, Theresia Degener, Anne Waldschmidt, and others is still largely unavailable to those who do not read German. Literature by contemporary German historians and disability studies scholars helps identify how racial hatred emerged *as a byproduct* of the conflation of systematic medical and nation-state ideologies—what G. K. Chesterton and Michael Perry referred to as the "evils of the scientific organized state" as early as 1929 (2000). The eugenics endeavor brought about international academic conferences (Black 2003, 70–71, 236, 245); academic appointments, courses, programs, majors, and departments in 376 universities across the United States (Cravens 1988, 53; D. Paul 1995, 10; Black 2003, 75); and global publication opportunities across Europe and North America (also infecting colonial geographies associated with the developed world). At the same time it *provided an additional rationale for disability genocide in Germany* as an active participant in the Eugenic Atlantic. It is both known and little understood that Germany came relatively late to the scientific sphere of eugenics (Weindling 1989, 7; Black 2003, 261). German scientists picked up legislative tactics, sterilization policies and practices, and the co-opting of institutions as research domains well *after* this kind of scientific empire building had taken place in France, Britain, the United States, Canada, and elsewhere. For instance, Lifton cites the admiration of Nazi doctors meeting at the University of Heidelberg in 1936 for American eugenicists, which they expressed by awarding an honorary doctorate to Harry Laughlin for his work on the development of sterilization laws and coercive institutionalization policies (2000, 40).

RACIAL DEVIANCE: INCAPACITIES OF ASSIMILATION To understand the dovetailing of racial and disability ideologies in the Eugenic Atlantic, we must begin with a discussion of the differences in the construction of these two social categories. In general, one might argue that an idea of biologically inferior bodies preceded the belief in a racially degraded body because Enlightenment science gave credence to the idea that bodies—like animal and plant species—could be classified based on their observed, "natural" characteristics.[2] For instance, as Zygmunt Bauman argues, "the father of scientific taxonomy, Linnaeus, recorded the division between the residents of Europe and inhabitants of Africa with the same scrupulous precision as that which he applied while describing the differences between crustacea and fishes" (2001b, 218). Linnaeus defined the "white" races through a celebratory referencing of their innate capacities "as inventive, full of ingenuity, orderly, and governed by laws," while "Negroes" were posed as their behavioral and cultural antitheses "endowed with all of the negative qualities which made them counterfoil for the superior race: they were regarded as lazy, devious, and unable to govern themselves" (ibid.). This contrast already demonstrates the degree to which racial marginalization depends on concepts of in-built biological inferiority (Fredrickson 2002, 1). Here we define "in-built inferiority" as those indelible characteristics responsible for the revelation of human variation, yet interpreted as unacceptable degrees of deviation. "Negroes" were not inferior with respect to debased cultural practices, but rather because their racial characteristics made them incapable of competing with the superior intelligence that presumably characterized Caucasian races (this is in direct accord with the definition of "feeblemindedness" proffered by eugenicists). European empiricism not only justified Caucasian superiority, but did so on the basis of biologies that were determined to be inherently deficient in their makeup.

Gesetz zur Verhütung

erbkranken Nachwuchses

vom 14. Juli 1933

mit Auszug aus dem Gesetz gegen gefährliche Gewohnheitsverbrecher
und über Maßregeln der Sicherung und Besserung vom 24. Nov. 1933

Bearbeitet und erläutert von

Dr. med. Arthur Gütt   Dr. med. Ernst Rüdin

Ministerialdirektor   o. ö. Professor für Psychiatrie an der Universität und Direktor
im Reichsministerium des Innern   des Kaiser Wilhelm-Instituts für Genealogie und Demographie
                                der Deutschen Forschungsanstalt für Psychiatrie in München

Dr. jur. Falk Ruttke

Geschäftsführer des Reichsausschusses für Volksgesundheitsdienst
beim Reichsministerium des Innern

Mit Beiträgen:

Die Eingriffe zur Unfruchtbarmachung des Mannes
und zur Entmannung
von Geheimrat Prof. Dr. med. Erich Lexer, München

Die Eingriffe zur Unfruchtbarmachung der Frau
von Geheimrat Prof. Dr. med. Albert Döderlein, München

Mit 15 zum Teil farbigen Abbildungen

J. F. Lehmanns Verlag / München 1934

TITLE PAGE OF «GESETZ ZUR VERHÜTUNG ERBKRANKEN NACHWUCHSES» (LAW FOR THE
PREVENTION OF PROGENY SUFFERING FROM A HEREDITARY DISEASE),
BY ARTHUR GÜTT, ERNST RÜDIN, AND FALK ALFRED RUTTKE (1934), AN EXPLICATION
OF THE LAW BASED ON THE U.S. "MODEL" POLICY WRITTEN BY EUGENICIST
HARRY LAUGHLIN (COURTESY OF WANSEE CONFERENCE HOUSE ARCHIVES)

Theories of race in the West grew steadily out of an argument about "stubborn particularities" that seemed to be the peculiar properties of isolated groups. Africans and Native Americans, for example, became synonymous in the Euro-American mindset with a primitive governing force of biology that made them incapable of assimilation at the level of culture. For much of the early colonial period, many racialized peoples were believed to embody a prior natural state with which the Caucasian race had lost contact. The "darker" peoples represented an unsullied, and therefore vulnerable, human nature, one that people could marvel at for its lack of modernity (that is, the extent to which it was "untouched" by civilized characteristics) and then could conquer on the basis of defining weaknesses. In many ways conquest, enslavement, and colonization of the New World can be interpreted as an exercise in the Caucasian races' domination of their own human "prehistory," projected onto the bodies of indigenous peoples of color. To early European explorers, inhabitants of the New World represented "children of the sun"—an infantilized yet desirable image of arrested human development prior to the demands and debacles of modernity in Europe. In other words, colonized peoples were consistently characterized as embodiments of a biological "prehistory," as throwbacks to an earlier moment in progressivist fantasies of the genus *Homo*. The conquest of racial Others provided the opportunity for European expansionists to retrieve an unspoiled, premodern version of an ever-complexifying Western self.

A principle of ingestion is at work in colonization, in which the conquering culture tries to internalize the features of the Other that it imagines as lacking in its own modern incarnation. The image of the "lazy, shiftless, and irresponsible" darker races living among abundant nature served as an approximation of what Euro-Americans felt they had surrendered in their rush to modernize. While the qualities associated with racialized peoples were castigated as "primitive" in the discourse of colonialism, the vehemence of their rejection stems from an ironic desire on the part of the colonizers to shed the complexity that presumably constituted their superiority. Like eugenicist renditions of the feebleminded, racialized Others presumably occupied a world equated with a less demanding past—one that required less agility, competency, and anxiety to navigate. They were also believed to occupy cultural locations where competition was either absent or significantly reduced, and thus, where there was less likelihood of disastrous military conflict and plagues born of overcrowding and scarce resources.

Yet, while colonial explorers and settlers believed they could return to an unsullied nature by taking possession of premodern lands and peoples, the indigenous inhabitants, in turn, were divested of the capacity to become "modern." In other words, European racism increasingly relied on the invention of culture as a unidirectional membrane where people of color remained forever located on the "primitive" side, while their Caucasian counterparts could partake of the best of both worlds. This division of racialized capacities as static qualities attributed to "less sophisticated" populations evidences what Adorno and Horkheimer have described as a "reduction to the natural, to sheer force, to that stubborn particularity which in the status quo constitutes the generality" (2000, 207). The capacity to assimilate, whether desirable or not as a population attribute, is the key quality stripped from those addressed by classifications of racial difference and, ultimately, disability as well. This "stubborn particularity" of a people becomes the site of recalcitrance to adaptation—not as a product of self-conscious, willed development, but rather as *an in-built incapacity* that cannot be transcended to any significant degree. For Adorno and Horkheimer, the "dialectical link" between "Enlightenment and domination" (ibid.) establishes authority by referencing categories of heredity, biology, and extracultural attributes as immutable characteristics of racialized identity.

In a slightly different vein, race scholars such as Mosse (2000) and Fredrickson (2002) have argued that European race hatred toward Jews develops from a belief in Jewish efforts to stubbornly sustain racial purity as a culture. While blacks remained "in their primitive state" (Mosse 2000, 201), Jews were feared to excel beyond the capacity of most Caucasian groups in modernity through their alignment in an anti-Semitic mindset with the newly reigning principles of "economic and monetary values" (Mosse 2000, 198). Thus, what Bauman (2001b) characterizes as the "pre-modern character of racism" becomes clear: a fear of modernization's demands on members of the dominant culture can be articulated with respect to another group's seeming lack of caution or inhibition with regard to them. Feeblemindedness was constituted in a similar formation, in which anxieties over modernization among nondisabled peoples were deflected (in an extreme form) onto those who were believed to occupy the category of "subnormality." While the "darker races" were viewed as insufficiently modern because of incapacities attributed directly to their racial makeup, Jewish peoples became despised as an adept intermediary between white and black. This interstitial position associated with Jewishness itself stemmed from arguments about some presumably innate lack of geographical and nationalist loyalties. While Jewish people, according to European racial science, shared common physiognomic and physical traits, they rejected an allegiance to the nation in favor of pure lines of filiation and religious community: "no matter how many great achievements the Jews were responsible for, they could not be absorbed into the European nations; they were not allowed to put down roots and so they were dismissed as rootless" (Adorno and Horkheimer 2000, 208). In other words, this imposed nomadic tendency of Jewish populations was misrecognized by even the most ardent proponents of racial purity in Europe as a quality that made Jews too "pure"—a hereditary predisposition that made them nonassimilable. While many late nineteenth- and early twentieth-century racial eugenicists argued that the success of nationalist groupings depended upon the ability to "maintain . . . purity and uniqueness of composition," Jewish "inability" to assimilate became an intractable and despised feature of a later named "racial" composition.[3]

Thus, one of the characteristics that connected African, Native American, and Jewish populations in the eugenics trajectory of racial particularity was a shared incapacity to assimilate. Although the biological qualities attributed to them differed, the "incapacity" to integrate, conjoined with historical associations of impurity (or excessive purity) and barbarity, marked all three racial groups as excessively deviant. A racial aberrancy that came to be consistently characterized as *biological*, rather than cultural, in nature: "racism proclaims that certain blemishes of a certain category of people cannot be removed or rectified—that they remain beyond the boundaries of reforming practices, and will do so for ever" (Bauman 2001b, 215). Such "incapacities" were presumed hereditary throughout the primary eugenics period. Biological arguments such as these point to a tendency "to emphasize the irreversibility and incurability of the damaging 'otherness' of the Other" (ibid., 214). This immutable quality attributed to races through biological traits serves as the primary locus for an analysis of human disqualification shared by racial Others *and* people with disabilities.

In other words, racial differences fell into a finite set of beliefs attributed to bodies marked as deterministically different by a dominant culture:

- A fear of insufficiency paradoxically conjoined with a desire to return to a lost nature projected by a dominant culture onto a minority culture
- A set of qualities attributable to cultural and environmental features but characterized as biological in origin
- The belief that the marked set of defective qualities may be "passed on" through reproduction, and thus, the perceived need to regulate procreation either through taboos against miscegenation or through social restrictions on the opportunity/ability to procreate within racial groups
- Prior stigmatized religious ascriptions of innate evil made legitimate by modern scientific empiricism
- The power of stigmatized differences causing the despised object's self-image to become increasingly depreciated and "at risk"
- Social engineering schemes involving radical segregation (for example,

Jim Crow laws or apartheid) and/or extermination practices toward groups considered inassimilable (not only the Holocaust, but also the Middle Passage or the removal of Native Americans to reservations)

- A utopian social vision of a future predicated upon participation of the dominant culture in a homogeneous cultural location where all undesirable embodiments are erased (for example, racist support of "back to Africa" movements in the United States and United Kingdom or the Nazi Madagascar Plan devised in pre–World War II Germany for the relocation of Jewish peoples)

The notion of a utopian social vision is critical because Western notions of modernity are bound up in utopian fantasies predicated on social drives toward perfected homogeneous communities—what Henri-Jacques Stiker refers to as the desire of the same (1999, 140). The attainment of this goal can only be evidenced by the successful ouster of historical differences that prove inherently contingent. Consequently, as with diagnostic regimes, an inherent principle of violence informs schemes developed around expunging undesirable biological variations identified as uniquely racial.

Disability studies brings to the discourse on the history of racism and racialized thinking the awareness that biological incapacities associated with racial traits are rarely recognized within the larger classifications of physical, sensory, and cognitive "defects" installed during this period. Race as a construct has been exclusively associated with a false projection of incapacity attributed to biological features. Within this formula, human incapacities are interpreted as exclusively racialized, which leads to a failure to recognize people with disabilities as the generic grouping referenced by presumably in-built physical, sensory, and cognitive "insufficiencies." In other words, our current theories of racial eugenics exclusively reference "race" as the social locus of ascribed insufficiency, while leaving disability as the default category of "real" human incapacity. This lack of address of disability eugenics in theories of racism ignores impairment as a socially mediated category of human difference and excludes discussion of the historical condition of disabled persons including disabled people of color. Similarly, the neglect of racial thinking in disability theory results in a problematic universalizing tendency that fails to account for differences in treatment across racial communities.

We believe that principles critiqued in racial eugenics can be paralleled by analyses of disability eugenics. Rather than allowing the two fields to develop on consistent yet separate grounds, we argue that the list of factors given above for the social construction of racism also applies to disability.

While disability has consistently been recognized as the one example of a "material" basis for human inequality, our argument is that race should be recognized as one key component of social disqualification based on an increasingly narrow continuum of human variation developed in the wake of the European Enlightenment. While the histories of Native Americans, African slaves, Jewish gentry, and disabled people are often historically and culturally distinct, the shared social marginality of these groups arises from the view of the "deviant" body as that which automatically disqualifies individuals from cultural participation (and biological desirability).

Our overriding effort is to demonstrate the ways in which disability came to be construed as a socially dehumanizing construct in tandem with theories of racial degeneracy. We recognize that this effort to draw parallels between race and disability is a risky enterprise in that race theories have sought to achieve "liberation" from dehumanizing constructs by distancing people of color from their association with the bearers of "more real" (or material) biological incapacities. We offer some ways in which racial discourse might avoid reifying people with disabilities as the bearers of "true" bodily deviance in their progressive social formulations, while also demonstrating the mutually beneficial value of analyses of race and disability in the repertoire of cultural criticism.

EUGENICS AS TRANSNATIONAL IDEOLOGY   The beliefs that informed racial and disability eugenics as peculiarly Western modes of intolerance toward biologically based differences explicitly dovetailed near the end of the eighteenth century. Eugenics as a transnational ideology developed the following characteristics:

- Interest in the possibility of "training" people with cognitive and physical differences as a core pursuit of scientific management techniques
- The rapid acceptance of confinement practices that sequestered massive numbers of disabled people and ethnic immigrants in institutions as available research populations
- The rise of hereditary theories of defect transmission that transformed disability from a familial or communal concern to a question of safeguarding and improving "public health" and national purity (later known as a country's hereditary pool or genetic stock)
- The invention of intelligence testing that expanded the category of defect from a primarily visible phenomenon manifested on or in the body to the measurement of an otherwise intangible, internal inferiority

- Restrictive public policies toward people with disabilities that limited or denied their participation in public institutions and privileges, such as marriage, reproduction, the labor market, the right to live in nonsegregated communities, and immigration

By restricting the social liberties and rights of disabled people, eugenics invented the category of "disability" that grouped people with widely divergent physical and cognitive characteristics under a single heading of "defect." While the generic grouping comprised proliferating subcategories of deviance, the consolidation of human variation under an exclusively derogatory classification imposed a disastrous logic of binary thinking. "Normal" and "feebleminded" (or "N" and "F," as eugenicists called the two groups) became the default categories for all human beings. The instruments for performing this classification scheme became increasingly complex and "sophisticated," but the power of eugenics lay in the relative simplicity of the formula. The transatlantic appeal of eugenics would rest primarily on its ability to offer up the power of classification to a host of professions and cultural administrators rather than hoarding the technology within a disciplinary or national domain. Such professions included nearly all of the disciplinary arenas that are today responsible for the management and oversight of people with disabilities, including medicine, therapy, charity, special education, social work, psychology, psychiatry, institutional administration, and policy.

The context for eugenics first took shape in France. In 1797 the capture in rural France of a "savage" or "wild boy," who reportedly could neither speak nor hear, led to his involuntary incarceration. During the period of his confinement the "wild boy" was objectified as a specimen of exhibition. French researchers pursued numerous efforts to "train" him out of his "prelinguistic" silence. Roger Shattuck (1980) has christened this objective most eloquently as "the forbidden experiment": "one that would reveal to us what 'human nature' really is beneath the overlays of society and culture" (41). These efforts began with the promise that bringing the "wild boy" to speech could provide the researchers with a passage back to their own lost primordial ancestry. The project was taken up by several renowned educators and physicians beginning with Sicard, who ran the Institute for Deaf-Mutes in Paris; Philippe Pinel, a celebrated physician of mental illness; and Jean-Marc Gastard Itard, a twenty-five-year-old medical student who became a close professional associate of Sicard's during the wild boy's stay (Shattuck 1980, 69). The responses of these professionals were quite various. Each characterized the boy as a "failure" in some respects. Sicard largely neglected him because

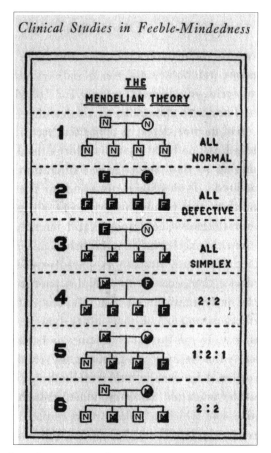

"NORMAL." AND "FEEBLEMINDED" PEDIGREE CHART, ILLUSTRATING MENDELIAN
HEREDITARY COMBINATIONS OF "DEFECT TRANSMISSION" (FROM DOLL 1917, 46)

of his responsibilities in running a large institution; Pinel declared him an "incurable idiot," in keeping with diagnostic nomenclature of the time; and Itard, who waged a bet with the first two that he could develop a successful training program, ultimately abandoned his rehabilitation project. According to Shattuck, Itard's program sought to accomplish five goals: to provide the boy with the ability to respond to others; to train his senses; to extend his physical and social needs; to teach him to speak; to teach him clear thinking (77). Among the practices used to train him were electrical shocks from a battery to signal bad behavior; naming him Victor because of his apparent attraction to the vowel sound *o*; and hanging the boy upside down from a fifth-story window to induce terror. While Itard reported enormous strides in

Victor's progress, he ultimately declared the experiment a failure because of the inordinate stress he placed on the ability to hear and speak.

Following on the heels of Itard's failed efforts to "civilize" Victor, the wild boy of Aveyron, Edouard Séguin argued for the systematic education of "fools and simpletons." Séguin's approach stressed rote repetition and the incremental discipline involved in gymnastics training. Those who were subject to this training regimen "suffered" from what Séguin referred to as an insufficient mastery of the will. "Idiocy," as he argued, stemmed from a defect of self-control where the basic skills of hygiene and motivation were lacking. The problem of "idiocy" could not be remedied without continuous surveillance and the oversight of institutions that would fill up one's days with activities that amounted to a performance of the social rituals that gave the domestic space of the middle class its familiar rhythms (what Foucault [1995, 249] refers to as the Tukes model of institutional discipline).

Like theories of racial primitives, "training" in separate institutional/educational sites recognized "idiocy" as a state of "infantilism" and "wildness" that could be overcome by modern disciplinary techniques. Gilroy refers to a parallel racial practice as "infrahuman blackness reconstituted in the 'half-devil, half-child' patterns favored by older colonial mentalities" (2001, 26). A series of sightings of "feral children" in Europe at this time harkened back to developed Western histories of kingdoms founded by "wolf children" abandoned or lost to human parenting communities. In addition to Victor, there were Young Peter the Wild Boy (found in Hanover, England, in 1726), Memmie Le Blanc (found in Champagne, France, in 1820), and Kasper Hauser (discovered in the streets of Nuremburg, Germany, in 1828). With the later addition of Kamala and Amala (found near Minapore, India, in 1920), all these cases represent "wild children" discovered during the primary eugenics period (Newton 2003). Such stories follow closely the tales of children "born of the beasts," such as the ancient Sumerian child Enkidu, or Romulus and Remus as the founders of Rome. Feral children exist on the border between human and animal but are then brought back into the civilizing fold of human society. As Michael Newton points out: "More strangely the same phrases [used to described other wild or feral children in history] are also used for those few children [today] who have lived through another perhaps crueler kind of loneliness, locked for years in solitary confinement in single rooms" (2003, xiii). Thus, feral children of the eighteenth and nineteenth centuries would comprise what contemporary behavioral sciences might classify as those with "severe behavior disorders." Akin to the colonized racial savage, the diagnosis of a feral child provided researchers with the possibility of access to a primitive stage of human development. If the "locked-in," presymbolic world of the feral child could be leveraged by the acquisition of language, then "defects" could be turned into an opportunity to recapture a time when human beings presumably still held a direct, unadulterated relationship to nature.

The bulk of this disciplinary regime at Séguin's institutional training sites sought to correct "behavioral aberrancy" by providing his subjects with a fully regimented daily routine, one that was orchestrated from dawn to dusk with tasks of self-care. Early training programs for "mental inferiors" sought to target the body and turn it into a tool of social manipulation. Like the various stories of feral children that abounded in the late eighteenth and early nineteenth centuries, the education of idiots would deliver its objects of intervention from their helplessness and "grotesque insufficiencies." Institutional "training" sought a way to rescue those classified as "idiots" from "mental darkness" (another rhetorical point of convergence between the Caucasian image of "darker peoples" and those with disability-based insufficiencies). The rhetoric of social rescue also parallels missionary efforts to deliver Christianity to "unenlightened" racial populations. In both cases, the presumed identification of inferior individuals corresponded to a dearth of access to modern belief systems equated with Euro-American civilization.

In 1848 Samuel Howe, director of the Perkins Institute for the Blind in Massachusetts, imported Séguin's techniques from France to the United States (1848, 19). Following Séguin, Howe subscribed to the theory of inferior will as the root cause of idiocy, but in his view the American brand of institutional training would not only salvage degraded lives but also relieve families of the burden of rearing "defectives" in the community. For Howe and other American disciples of the French school, "idiots" were not just incapable of helping themselves but also threatened the fabric of society. Family attention to other, "healthy" children was reduced because of the excessive demands of "idiots" on parental energies. Further, the family's need to attend to the "idiot" upset the country's industrializing labor pool by preventing at least one parent from working. Finally, "idiots" also proved a menace to communities by exposing "normal" children to the inappropriate behaviors of those who lacked the capacity to censor their own actions. U.S. adherents of training schools for idiocy repeated many of the practices of the French while further steeping educators, institutional administrators, and the public in the newly christened philosophy and typology of "defectives."[4] Eugenics documents reference Séguin's teachings in an almost obligatory fashion as justification for American practices.

While institutions of various kinds, such as asylums, were common in much of Europe, the practice of institutionalizing citizens on the basis of faulty biology was relatively new. To "sell" such a practice, proponents of education for idiots promised institutionalized training as a temporary intervention; institutional advocates argued that those identified as eligible for training would be removed from the community only so long as it took to train them for a life of normalcy. Institutions reassured communities and families that once training was complete, the newly rehabilitated subject would be returned to pursue a life of independence to whatever degree possible. This promise of return played a key role in efforts to convince skeptical legislatures, and the public at large, that training schools were progressive rather than punitive operations. Within ten years European and U.S. institutions began to transform themselves from educational to custodial structures, and training missions quickly gave way to efforts of social erasure for "undesirables" (Rothman 1971, 265).

The nineteenth-century British scientist Sir Francis Galton is credited with coining the term *eugenics*.[5] But by his day custodial practices in institutions for the feebleminded (the catchall term for this era's many-faceted diagnoses of defect) already evidenced an increasingly restrictive approach to those identified as "inferior." While a theory of heredity gave scientific support for the formal exclusion of disabled people from mainstream social life, training schools were the setting for the formulation of a new diagnostic classification ("idiots," then "the feebleminded," and later "the subnormal"). Once an impetus for segregating citizens, however temporarily, was in place, it was only a minor transition to permanent incarceration. In the guise of a liberal sentiment (care for those who could not care for themselves), eugenics took shape as an educational rescue mission for children who were seen as exhibiting signs that would make then unworthy of education (from atrophied muscles to crossed eyes to delayed acquisition of reading skills). Institutional administrators, trainers, and later, psychiatrists/psychologists soon recognized the institution as an ideal laboratory with a ready-made research population, and from then on, institutions for the feebleminded sought to retain their charges. Among U.S. eugenicists Henry H. Goddard argued this point most baldly: "We need to study them very seriously and very thoroughly; we need to hunt them out in every possible place and take care of them" (1916, 9). Advertisements were issued in professional eugenics journals such as *Psycho-asthenics* that sought to appeal to researchers, promising them nice laboratories and a ready-made population for experimentation. At the same time that an in-house disability research business escalated, with the promise of careers for young professionals, institutional administrators began acknowledging that "it was not expedient to return to the community a certain number of the cases who had received all the instruction the school had to offer" (Fernald 1893, 210).

The widely circulated popular journals, medical articles, and pamphlet publications of the eugenics era show how the rhetoric of institutionalization changed from training those who were determined to be immobile "idiots" for some self-care and independence, to dealing with the social menace represented by feebleminded individuals—that is, anyone displaying marks or signs of nonnormalcy as broadly conceived but particularly those diagnosed with both physical and cognitive disabilities. Unlike its French and British counterparts, American eugenics increasingly emphasized the relationship of physical "stigmata" to cognitive inferiority and in doing so, provided mechanisms for analyzing the visible surface of the body as an indicator of an otherwise intangible interior defect (Monroe 1897, 7).

Thus, the tethering of physical and cognitive disability in the shared cultural locations of disability across the Eugenic Atlantic came to be articulated as a fait accompli, and juxtaposition helped to round out a picture of human defectives as inferior in every aspect of their humanity. The importance of this connection between physical and cognitive disability cannot be underestimated because most studies of eugenics have continued to reproduce the mistaken notion that the category of "the feebleminded" referred to cognitive impairments alone. Eugenicists recognized that the drastic measures planned for disabled bodies would need to be presented by stripping away as many human attributes as possible—specifically, as in the case of racial populations, by turning disabled people into biologies deprived of sentience.[6] The object of institutionalization was constituted through a form of scientific double jeopardy: as disabled individuals found themselves shrouded in the debasing language of "burden," "menace," and "defect," the probability of finding themselves *permanently* incarcerated increased. Thus, the constitution of the disabled object—those whom we refer to as members of the "subnormal nation"—led to its acceptable eternal sequestration, while sequestration resulted in an increasing lack of public familiarity with disability as a sign of persistent human variation. As familiarity lessened and eugenics rhetoric further debased its clientele, Eugenic Atlantic attitudes toward disability grew increasingly less tolerant of human differences. Thus, the multinational conversation in eugenics cultivated a triangular cultural space (akin to the geometric depiction of the slave trade) that scientifically reconfirmed the debasement of biologically based differences.

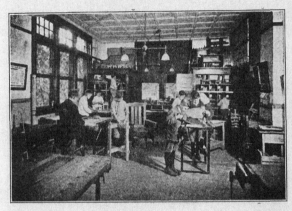

THE TRAINING SCHOOL
- - *AT* - -
VINELAND NEW JERSEY

Devoted to the interests of those whose minds have not
developed normally

Established in 1888---For the study, care and training
of mentally deficient children over five years of age,
who are clean in their personal habits. The tuition
rate is $75 a month.

Research Laboratories---Thoroughly equipped School
Department.

C. EMERSON NASH, *Superintendent.*

E. R. JOHNSTONE, *Director.*

ADVERTISEMENT FOR THE VINELAND TRAINING SCHOOL/LABORATORY IN NEW JERSEY
(FROM «JOURNAL OF PSYCHO-ASTHENICS» 25 [SEPTEMBER 1920–JUNE 1921])

Additionally, eugenicists achieved their goals through a carefully orchestrated public relations campaign that recognized the rhetoric of disability as
a critical precursor to increasingly lethal policies. As one surveys eugenics literature of the period, it becomes evident that approaches to disabled people
that were initially unspeakable—permanent institutionalization, marriage
laws, immigration laws, sterilization laws, and, eventually, even extermination—gradually creep into the discourse as a whispered plausibility. And
once a radical management strategy was articulated—even as an intervention that the general public would not tolerate—it took only a matter of a
few years for the unspeakable possibility to come to fruition. The eugenics

literature shows how the vocalization of "impossible" solutions facilitates the realization of the most drastic interventions. Once the unspeakable is spoken, to resignify African American novelist Toni Morrison's phrase, the road is already paved for that very impossibility to become reality.

As a transatlantic scientific movement, eugenics bound much of Europe and North America in a concerted movement to rid disabilities from a country's national spaces. The improvement of genetic stock was not merely an internal program undertaken by a variety of nations at the same time, but rather a cultural traffic in the cultivation of a shared distaste toward "deviance" and unacceptable human variations. For instance, when the Second International Congress of Eugenics was held in 1921 at the American Museum of Natural History in New York, the event attracted more than three hundred international delegates from Belgium, Denmark, England, France, Italy, Norway, and Sweden. With memories of World War I still fresh, Germany and Russia were excluded even though professional ties remained strong and cordial.

Both the British and French played a strong role in eugenics through conference organization and attendance, professional and popular publishing, and national policy influence. Although the French Eugenics Society had only slightly more than a hundred members at its peak, it sent the largest number of delegates from any country to the first and second eugenics congresses. In addition, the international prestige of its members, coupled with the key role of France in the origins of eugenics, allowed the French delegates to exert significant influence over areas of policy and publishing in the field (Schneider 2002, 277). As eugenics gained steam, European and North American nations cited each other as reinforcement for restrictive policy implementation. The French referenced and sought to emulate the work of Karl Pearson at the University of London and that of Charles Davenport at Cold Spring Harbor Laboratory, Long Island, New York (Schneider 2002, 276). The British eugenics movement, spearheaded largely after Galton's death in 1911 by physician Robert Rentoul, drew directly upon U.S. eugenics policy. In his 1903 pamphlet advocating the adoption of sterilization policies in Britain, Rentoul relied significantly on summaries of parallel policies developed in Minnesota, Colorado, Wisconsin, and other U.S. states (Black 2003, 208). After its inception in 1908, the Eugenics Education Society in Britain had little to do but adopt American attitudes toward negative eugenics because of a dearth of eugenics-based research. Yet, in spite of a variety of American-style eugenics advocates, Britain developed its own brand of eugenics. For example, no sterilization law was ever successfully passed in Great Britain, and coercive approaches such as marriage restriction and compulsory segregation did not become formal government policies. As Richard Soloway (1990) has argued, "[British] eugenicists were more adept at influencing other groups and individuals and at reinforcing 'eugenic tendencies' where they found them than they were at establishing a clear, dominant role for themselves and their movement" (xiii). Just as in France, most eugenic efforts in Britain coalesced around the implementation of positive eugenic practices that addressed specific concerns over declining birth rates.

Nevertheless, each nation referenced other countries' "successes" in eugenics legislation and research practices as a means to keep pressure on legislatures, scientific communities, and the general public with respect to support for repressive practices toward disabled people. In numerous instances the scientific community in one country celebrated the successes in another to bolster its own efforts. The transatlantic commerce in restrictive disability measures provides one of the earliest examples of a cross-cultural scientific discourse based on a shared proving ground of the unacceptability of named disability attributes. Most nations in the Eugenic Atlantic cultivated an extranational stigma against individuals with a variety of conditions: environmentally borne illnesses, such as tuberculosis; congenital conditions, such as club foot and "cretinism"; sensory differences, such as deafness and blindness; cognitive processing differences; and psychiatric conditions, such as schizophrenia and acute depression. Disabled people embodied differences considered so impairing that the denial of their humanity paved the way for the murderous policies implemented in Germany in the 1930s and 1940s.

THE NAZI EUTHANASIA MOVEMENT, 1933–1945 From the passage of the first German sterilization law in 1933, which was based directly on the U.S. sterilization law for defectives, to the end of 1945, the Nazi government oversaw the systematic destruction of disabled German citizens (Proctor 1988, 101). The campaign to kill "lives unworthy of life" began simultaneously with the construction of concentration/work camps. Studies of this period have often overlooked the fact that the killing technologies used in the death camps were first developed and implemented on the bodies of disabled people, many of whom had been incarcerated within psychiatric institutions. The reasons for this neglect of disabled people's history in modern Germany are multifaceted, reflecting both a paucity of historical information on the subject and a continuing social reluctance to imagine disability as a valued aspect of the human biological continuum. In addition, until recently the lack of a socially based analysis of disability has left this constituency mired in models of pathos and tragedy developed and implemented during the eugenics era.

Recent scholarship has helped to establish a pattern of violence against disabled people perpetuated by the Nazis during World War II that proves consistently in line with Eugenic Atlantic thinking. Disabled German citizens were evaluated for extermination, and Nazi troops targeted incarcerated populations of disabled people in psychiatric institutions in Austria, Poland, Prussia, and Czechoslovakia to "clear space" in these buildings for the establishment of military headquarters (Proctor 1988, 189; Burleigh 1994, 130–34; H. Friedlander 1997, 158). The destruction of disabled people resulted from the implementation of an oppressively narrow conception of human value based on aesthetic criteria and also functioned as a means to create more "room and resources" for the sought-after proliferation of the healthy Germanic *Volk*. Like eugenics proper, such murderous campaigns were performed under the guises of "mercy" and economic utility. If disability robbed one of a viable life, reasoned Nazi eugenicists, then destruction was for their own benefit, and that of the nation, through the alleviation of "suffering" and a lessening of institutionalization as a burden upon the national economy.

The euthanasia campaign began with the murder of disabled children by starvation and lethal injection during the mid- to late 1930s (H. Friedlander 1997, 39). Since there was little public protest against such actions, the program was expanded to include those diagnosed with such conditions as epilepsy, physical "malformation," insanity, feeblemindedness, depression, and alcoholism, to name just a few (H. Friedlander 1997, 76; Burleigh 1994, 184–87). All these conditions were thought to be heritable, and German eugenics, extending the lead of American, French, and British science, espoused the belief that a superior race of people could be engineered by the eradication of "defectives." These people were seen as parasites upon the German state due to their apparent lack of utility as laborers. For instance, Proctor cites English and German sources of the period arguing that "Negroes" should not be killed because they represented a valuable labor force, while disabled people were financial burdens on the state whose deaths would benefit the nation (1988, 179). (Of course, this point overlooks the mortality that always accompanies slave systems, particularly for human chattel who become disabled as a result of inhumane labor and living conditions or for those killed after being born with a disability on slave plantations.) Yet, unlike other participants in the ideology of the Eugenic Atlantic, Germany developed one of the most advanced and robust rehabilitation regimes, which ultimately surpassed anything in the rest of Europe or the United States (H. Friedlander 1997, 157; Vogt 2002, 39–40). The reigning belief was that the government would do everything possible to return each citizen to the work force. However, those who "failed" their rehabilitation program found themselves permanently excluded from categories of citizenship. In this sense, one sees a critical link between the depth of state commitments to rehabilitation as the promise of disability erasure and the sedimentation of a "nonremediable," lower tier of subhumanity preparatory to irreversible segregation and extermination.

By October 1939 Hitler had signed the order (backdated to 1 September to coincide with the beginning of the war) for the T4 program, which commenced the systematic killing of citizens with discernible disabilities (H. Friedlander 1997, 67). As a pointedly "liberal" turn on the part of the Nazis, disabled veterans, dynamic disabled laborers, and the elderly were to be exempted, with the accompanying hope that the segregation and erasure of other disabled people would pass with little remark by concerned families, churches, and citizens (H. Friedlander 1997, 81–82; Aly, Chroust, and Pross 1994, 44). Scholars of Nazi public health have argued that the medical profession, accompanied by its bureaucracies and processing measures, permitted euthanasia to occur with little protest, and that once public outcry seemed incontestable, killing methods could continue in a decentralized fashion by medical practitioners who believed that they were doing the right thing for "afflicted" people and the nation (Bauman 2001b, 94).

Although nearly every German hospital participated in the euthanasia killing programs (primarily through the use of lethal injection and starvation), there were six primary killing centers: Brandenburg, Grafeneck, Hadamar, Bernburg, Sonnenstein, and Hartheim Castle (Proctor 1988, 191; Aly, Chroust, and Pross 1994, 39; H. Friedlander 1997, 89). In each of these institutions the Nazis constructed an elaborate technology of murder that included a processing procedure that falsified death records; a gas chamber for the "efficient" execution of many individuals at one time; an autopsy room for the advancement of medical "knowledge" and the lucrative extraction of gold teeth; a body stacking room; and, finally, crematoria ovens (H. Friedlander 1997, 93–98; Snyder and Mitchell 2002). This system of murder was the basis for later practices used against racial, ethnic, and sexual minorities in the death camps—a clear link between disability and other minority identities. The psychiatric killings in particular served as the foundation for the "final solution" in that relocation schemes such as the Madagascar Project informed most approaches to the "Jewish problem" before the

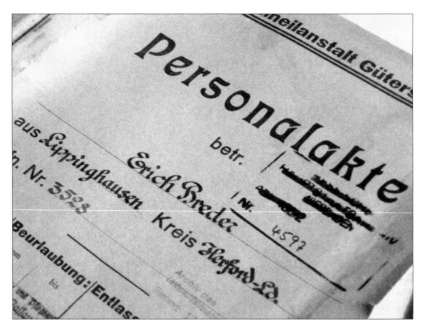

T4 INSTITUTIONAL FILE FOR "EUTHANASIA" VICTIM (COURTESY OF
HADAMAR PSYCHIATRIC INSTITUTION ARCHIVE)

successful implementation of institutional gas chambers (Lifton 2000, 76; Bauman 2001b, 105–6). In addition, the improved "efficiency" of the psychiatric killings led Nazi officials to imagine the possibility of the extermination of millions by the end of World War II (H. Friedlander 1997, 301). When killing centers completed the eradication of disabled individuals, apparatus such as the crematoria ovens were dismantled and sent off for reuse at the newly constructed death camps (Snyder and Mitchell 2002). Also, many medical personnel who operated the gas chambers in psychiatric institutions were transferred to oversee the ethnic cleansing operations (Lifton 2000, 134–42).

The human and cultural aftermath of the Nazi euthanasia campaign was devastating. While the liberation of concentration camps rescued thousands of survivors on the brink of starvation and extermination, there was no corresponding event of this scale at psychiatric institutions. The euthanasia campaign proved so successful that few institutional residents remained. The killing of disabled people by the earlier methods of lethal injection and starvation continued during the "wild euthanasia period" even after the surrender of Germany to Allied troops (Burleigh 1994, 261–63; H. Friedlander 1997, 162). Ultimately more than 240,000 disabled individuals were murdered (see

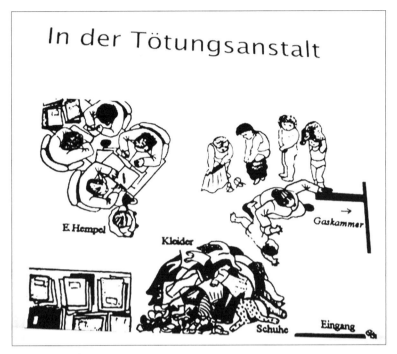

SURVIVOR'S RENDITION OF CHILDREN BEING SENT TO THE GAS CHAMBER, 1945
(COURTESY OF BRANDENBURG PSYCHIATRIC INSTITUTION COMMEMORATIVE EXHIBIT)

table 1 for totals from 1940–41). Today entire populations of disabled people (such as the many polio survivors who contribute to disability studies thinking and activism in the United States and the United Kingdom) are largely absent from the contemporary German landscape. Physicians who participated in the euthanasia campaign (but not in concentration camps) have never been successfully prosecuted because the line between medicine and murder fails to be articulated. The murder of disabled people, unlike the killing of ethnic and sexual Others, has continued to go unrecognized as a crime against humanity, except in the eyes of a handful of intellectuals and activists.

CONCLUSION: DISABILITY AS MASTER TROPE OF HUMAN DISQUALIFICATION The systematic extermination of disabled and racialized peoples at the end of the Eugenic Atlantic era allows for a juxtaposition of the intertwined fate of two populations that share an identification as biologically "subhuman." If we consider racism to be tethered to an absolutist formulation of biology, as most racism scholars now suggest, then drawing parallels between racism and ableism seem not only plausible

Table 1. Killings at German psychiatric centers, 1940–41

Center	Victims in 1940	Victims in 1941	Total
Grafeneck	9,839	Closed	9,839
Brandenburg	9,772	Closed	9,772
Hartheim	9,670	8,599	18,269
Sonnenstein	5,943	7,777	13,720
Bernburg	Not yet open	8,601	8,601
Hadamar	Not yet open	10,072	10,072
Total	35,224	35,049	70,273

Source: H. Friedlander 1997, 109.

but necessary—especially since disability in post-Enlightenment thought is located within a conception of degraded biology. Because "disability" designates individuals rather than groups, the technical usage of racism as that which marks a group may not seem to apply. However, the intertwined histories outlined here, from quests for racial purity to eugenics campaigns to rid human "defects" from the biological continuum to the systematic extermination efforts of the Holocaust, seem to suggest that the two terms may be situated in a much more intimate lineage, even though disability has been traditionally situated outside of race as group identity based on shared somatic characteristics. Skin pigmentation, religious practices, cultural separatism, and refusals to assimilate came to be viewed by the dominant culture as signs of deterministic incapacity and therefore provided a basis for exclusion. As Celeste Langan (2001) points out, disability is a "transient stigmatizing identity" and refuses a more static cultural assignment based on generic features (465).

Yet socially marked bodies were still cross-referenced in public hygiene movements that characterized Eugenic Atlantic thinking in order to demonstrate race as an indicator of abject, unbearable ("disabled") bodies. Diagnoses were sometimes used to isolate distinct tribes or "species" of humans, such as "Mongoloid idiots" or "the Tubercular" or "Blind idiots," but a general category of otherness, such as "the unfit," seems to have suited civic goals, collecting multiple diagnoses and rare "disorders" as those destined for "special treatment." In this sense, one might think of disability as "the master trope of human disqualification" (Mitchell and Snyder 2000, 3). To successfully malign a socially stigmatized identity, it is not enough, as George Fredrickson has argued, to enact a "group centered prejudice and snobbery"; instead, such antipathy must be expressed "with a single mindedness and brutality that go far beyond a marked 'heterophobia'" (2002, 1). Ultimately, this socially realized "brutality" can be characterized as the product of widely shared ableist assumptions that disqualify groups of people based upon what is characterized as a biologically coded insufficiency: "we might say racism exists when one ethnic group or historical collectivity dominates, excludes, or seeks to eliminate another on the basis of differences that it believes are hereditary and unalterable" (Fredrickson 2002, 170). If we refer to this stigmatizing referencing strategy as ableism, then we arrive at that which is most shared (rather than distinctive) about modes of modern prejudice often identified only by analyses and studies of "race" as a biological fallacy of one's predecessors or a lingering "bad idea."

It is not coincidental that the policies that hemmed in racialized groups in Europe and the United States paralleled legislation promoted by eugenicists against people with disabilities. Legalized discrimination, which characterizes the existence of a racist regime, finds its correlatives in the policies that reflect eugenics discourses on disability: Marriage restriction laws against people with cognitive disabilities, coerced sterilization, routine institutionalization, mandated segregation in schools, class-based communities of the homeless, sheltered workshops, and farm colonies all make up a social landscape occupied by those designated as existing at the bottom rungs of social ladders of being. That such policies have characterized life for people of color and disabled people in the West provides an opportunity to rethink the extent to which social marginalization is dependent upon tropes of bodily based deviancy. As Back and Solomos have argued, race comes to be increasingly "coded as culture" by the twentieth century in that "the central groups are fixed, made natural, confined within a pseudo-biologically defined culturalism" (2000, 18–19). We might also shift their emphasis slightly in order to argue that race becomes coded as culturalism to the degree that it overlaps with the discourses of disability that define modern strategies of marginalization based on insurmountable bodily insufficiencies. In other words, a distinctive feature of modernity can be traced in the development of disability as the preeminent sign of other culturally despised identities.

Our emphasis upon the cross-national characteristics of these marginalizing strategies is not meant to overlook the differences that exist within various nation-states' particular responses to their own subordinated communities, but rather to highlight the history of eugenics as a transatlantic phenomenon. Rather than sustain race and disability as separate phenomena within eugenics, we identify a convergence that condemns stigmatized groupings to a shared, deterministic fate. That the systematic killing of Jews, Romany, and gay peoples in the Holocaust was devised in the gas chambers of the psychiatric killing hospitals provides an instructive parable for future research. Disability as the master trope of human disqualification in modernity prefaces

an understanding of inassimilable racial and ethnic differences by providing an empirical designation for "unfit" bodies. Like discourses of national
differences that, in turn, support investments in absolutist racial differences,
disability may provide a key to the recognition of an underlayer of classification systems based on disqualifying bodily traits that jettison certain people
from inclusion in the continuum of acceptable human variations.

The vision of the Eugenic Atlantic achieved, first and foremost, the proliferation of the belief that certain groups in society "are so despised or disparaged that the upholders of the norms feel compelled to make them exceptions to the promise or realization of equality, they can be denied the
prospect of equal status only if they allegedly possess some extraordinary deficiency that makes them less than fully human" (Fredrickson 2002, 12). The
important parallels between disability and racialized forms of discrimination
can be witnessed in this quotation, which was intended to characterize the
distinctive contours of racism itself. Yet one need only insert "disability" as
the sentence's referent to recognize that such claims also prove true for people with disabilities, because nearly all theorists of modern racism locate the
origins of formalized racism in the cultural groundwork of disability (that is,
in-built biological inferiority).

Thus, like racism, disability as a formalized classification of disqualification develops in the wake of the European Enlightenment, when Western
societies began to move from the designation of social Others based on religious intolerance to marginalizing practices based on theories of biologically
based insufficiencies. Within the former system of discrimination, religious
conversion was held out as a promise of acceptance for ideological deviants;
within the latter system no promise of assimilation was offered, since the
system was based on the notion of deficiencies that cannot be overcome.
As Zygmunt Bauman has argued, the belief in a liberated individualism depends on drawing an "arbitrary dividing line between norm and abnormality" (2001b, 28). In a "social democratic space open to everyone," those who
cannot effectively participate are excluded on the basis of their own bodily
failings. The realization of equality is constituted right at the moment when
bodies that harbor extraordinary deficiencies are made to appear as nonremediable. Thus, those exterminated as unproductive in Fascist Germany were
only condemned once the state had offered them the most modern and vigorous rehabilitation program it could devise. The fault for those who failed
to meet that objective was then safely located within them rather than in the
wider social system of supports.

The Eugenic Atlantic produced racial and disability doctrines premised on a uniquely modern utopian fantasy of a future world uncontaminated by defective bodies—either disabled, racialized, or both at the same time (see our documentary video, *A World without Bodies* [2002]). Either through intensified and state-sanctioned reproductive restrictions imposed on the right of "defective" bodies to procreate or through efforts to systematically exterminate undesirables, semiproductives, and nonassimilables once and for all, the modern states of the Eugenic Atlantic aimed to purify otherwise distinctive collectivities of a shared social menace. Their commonality was marked not in the likenesses of their valued citizens, but rather in the existence of a common social dis-ease with the biologically stigmatized. In this way racialized and disabled Others were catapulted to the status of transatlantic pariahs.

Part II

ECHOES

OF

EUGENICS

FOUR

After the Panopticon | *Contemporary Institutions as Documentary Subject*

The body no longer has to be marked; it must be trained and re-trained; its time must be measured out and fully used; its forces must be continually applied to labor.

MICHEL FOUCAULT, "PUNITIVE SOCIETY"

This chapter analyzes parallels between Michel Foucault's research into disciplinary regimes in the nineteenth century and the sequestration of objectionable bodies in institutionalization practices of today. We focus upon those practices as recorded in a recent series of documentary films by Frederick Wiseman, taped on location at the Helen Keller Institute for the Deaf and Blind in Talladega, Alabama. In works such as *Madness and Civilization* (1988b), *The Birth of the Clinic* (1975), and *Discipline and Punish* (1995) Foucault identifies key European sites, such as the asylum, the courts, the prison, the clinic, and educational facilities, that adopted shared techniques of discipline. These techniques revolved around tools that labeled, partitioned, and scrutinized bodies in order to exact noncorporeal compliance, which referenced subjectivities rather than physical bodies as the locus of intervention. In the attempt to establish these systems of compliance, Foucault's cultural locations all become sites where pathology is meted out in order to make bodies "legible" and thus productive. To accomplish this task institutions increasingly looked to pathologizing professions, such as medicine, psychiatry, and ultimately, rehabilitation, for expert testimony that transformed the "monsters" of an earlier time into "abnormals." This critical shift, for Foucault, signaled a naturalization of difference that placed it on a continuum of human capacities. Consequently, in a uniquely Foucauldian turn, the power of human difference was essentially domesticated and stripped of its ability to reference the power of alterity. Ironically, then, monstrosity's potential as a source of agency was diminished and one might read the rise of cultural forms such as the freak show as nostalgia for a less neutralized expression of difference.

Our brief overview of Foucault's analyses is drawn in part from his lectures as collected in *Abnormal* (2003), where the domestication of the disabled body's potentially powerful difference is explicitly addressed. While his other works focus on the pathologization of sexuality, criminality, gender, childhood, and the lower classes, *Abnormal* explicitly addresses disabled bodies and, particularly, the rise of eugenics. One great frustration for disability scholars had been the glaring lack of direct analysis about disability in Foucault's work, although his insights have proven eminently useful for an analysis of disability. With the exception of *Abnormal*, Foucault's most important works on the history of pathologization consistently arrive on the doorstep of eugenics only to stop short. Much of his work intends to explain how Western societies inevitably arrived at eugenic practices as the quintessential expression of modernity. Eugenics occupies an almost deterministic lineage in the Foucauldian history of Western development. Consequently, the publication of *Abnormal* was welcomed as filling an important gap in Foucault's work.

We seek to understand the ways in which a Foucauldian analysis of docile bodies still operates in contemporary institutions as a historical remnant of outdated carceral regimes. Although Foucauldian concepts of governmentality might appear most applicable to the contemporary management of disability—the dissemination of norms of acceptable behaviors and appearances outside of imprisoning walls—our parallel of Foucault and Wiseman focuses on bodies still embedded within incarcerating settings. The cultural justification for continuing institutionalization as an approach to disability occurs strictly on the basis of physical, sensory, and cognitive differences recognized as nonintegrable. In part, our effort here is to show that some disabled bodies—particularly those that Wiseman's films identify as "multi-handicapped"—exist within punitive regimes that harken back to a seemingly antiquated mode of state power. This is important because today's nursing homes, sheltered workshops, and twenty-four-hour-care facilities all function in a way that we might associate with a more *barbaric* historical moment of treatment for bodies deemed excessively aberrant. Their euphemistic names suggest "kinder and gentler" institutional regimes that Foucault might have analyzed with his usual zeal and rightful disdain. Yet these contemporary carceral facilities also reference some uniquely current approaches to the management of deviancy and the specific forms of resistance that they conjure up. These existing cultural locations of disability prove significant as sites of analysis in that they simultaneously remind us of a past that we believed we had superseded and gesture toward a future that we need to avoid.

THE END(S) OF EUGENICS   Like Foucault's historical research, Wiseman's films seek out many of the cultural locations typically occupied by disabled people: prisons, hospitals, charity networks, sheltered workshops, resident facilities, and vocational training structures. While neither theorist nor documentary filmmaker situates himself as an analyst of disability explicitly, their methodological approaches provide important insight into the structures and rationale of modern incarceration practices—particularly for those imprisoned as a result of some organic, "in-built inferiority."

As we have shown, both the United States and Europe participated in the practice of removing disabled people from participation as citizens. In the process, eugenics-based practices forwarded a language of training that justified disabled people's sequestration; debased the clientele in order to further secure their exclusion from the rights and privileges of the majority of society; sought to physically restrict them from opportunities to procreate; shifted their representation in the dominant culture from misfortune to menace; and pursued research programs based on the existence of a population so alienated from their rights as citizens that their consent was unnecessary.

This chapter attempts to discern the echoes of eugenic practices in contemporary U.S. society. While the term *eugenics* gradually became ineffectual as a banner beneath which professionals were willing to march, the movement's influence was sweeping and profound. Although eugenics may have lost its power to galvanize research and institutional rationale, this alone does not imply the loss of its influence. While most scholars of eugenics have tended to claim that the movement collapsed in reaction to Nazi atrocities during World War II, this argument strikes us as inadequate to explain the toppling of such a developed cultural edifice. The image of eugenics as a tree whose roots grow deep into the earth and draw sustenance from a vast range of fields—anatomy, biology, medicine, psychiatry, surgery, statistics, anthropology, sociology, statistics, education, religion, economics, politics, geography, history—suggests that it would not be felled so easily.

It remains to be proven that news of Nazi atrocities—particularly against disabled people—was ever adequately circulated by the Western press to dismantle the influence of eugenics so absolutely. Rather, we suggest that the movement had run its course with respect to its primary function as a public policy campaign with scientific justifications. By the beginning of World War II, eugenics had accomplished (though in a somewhat less sweeping form than its practitioners had hoped) nearly everything it had set out to accomplish in both the policy and public opinion arenas. By initiating legislation at both the state and federal levels, such as marriage laws, immigration laws, coerced institutionalization, mandatory sterilization, and even physical eradication (in Germany), the eugenics movement had largely achieved its aims. In addition, the definition of "subnormal" had become so vast and fluid that those who were potentially threatened with inclusion beneath its umbrella of inferiority must have grown increasingly anxious. The movement's success led to its demise (or, perhaps, its lack of further utility). Like other disciplinary movements that once made up the primary root system of eugenics, such as the community mental health movement in psychology, eugenics proper found its singular authority challenged. Yet, in keeping with our chosen metaphor, the trunk of eugenics may have shriveled, but its disciplinary roots continued to thrive in the ideologies and practices that gave eugenics momentum for more than fifty years. Eugenics thinking and methodologies had infused the cultural locations of disability to such an extent that a study of the period allows us to better detect the ongoing undercurrents that once fed the formal movement.

This chapter focuses on one such site—an institution for the "multi-handicapped"—in order to gauge the degree to which eugenics beliefs and practices continue in our own period. Methods of discipline, more than punishment, sit at the heart of contemporary institutions, and they inevitably draw their power from techniques established in the late eighteenth and nineteenth centuries. It was during this period, as Foucault's research makes clear, that the target of power shifted from the physical body to the mind of the disciplined subject. This historical shift is key to comprehending the organization of contemporary institutional life to which Wiseman's films give us access.[1]

We will begin with an overview of Wiseman's Deaf-Blind documentary series as a pathway for addressing the place of disability in his oeuvre. Part

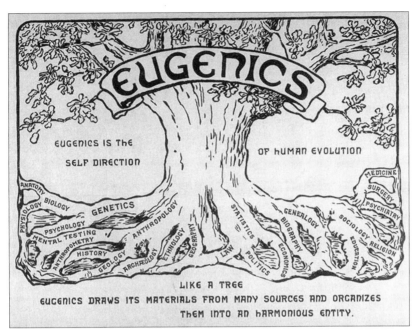

EUGENICS AS A TREE, WITH ROOTS IN MANY DISCIPLINES, AN IMAGE THAT FED INTO THE
CULTIVATION OF EUGENICS AS A HEGEMONIC DISCIPLINARY FORMATION
(COURTESY OF THE SMITH ELY JELLIFFE EUGENICS COLLECTION)

of this discussion involves a brief return to some of our previously discussed historical coordinates of disability history; particularly since it was these traditions that led to the latter twentieth-century practice of separating disabilities into primarily orthopedic or cognitive classifications. This diagnostic practice provides part of the background for Wiseman's work. From there we move to an analysis of North American institutional contexts as they developed in the nineteenth century. In doing so, we use Foucault's analysis of disciplinary structures to expand on our discussions in chapter 1 of David Rothman's history of U.S. asylums.

In part, this history depends upon revisiting the ways in which early nineteenth-century treatment programs metamorphosed from rehabilitative to custodial institutions within a single decade. Concepts of custodialism return us to Foucault's concept of modern "docile bodies." Foucault's later work may have moved away from the analysis of institutional contexts and toward a wider cultural application of discipline (though he does argue that *The Order of Things* extends the case study work of *Madness and Civilization*). Our own analysis will return us to foundational institutional sites and contemporary custodial and training practices as depicted in Wiseman's films. While avoiding arguments for a direct line of transmission between Foucault and Wiseman, our discussion of the latter's documentary techniques demonstrates a parallel methodology informing both approaches. In a basic sense, and by taking the guide that archaeology unearths which Wiseman's editing discloses, sifting through the dailies and the moments for indicative sites of resistance, both expose the underpinnings of coercion as the subtle and pervasive maneuvers of power that emerge in the act of classifying and renaming kinds of deviance in the cultural locations of disability.

MULTI-HANDICAPPED   During the mid-1980s, Wiseman produced a four-part series of films that sought to record the operations of institutions in Talladega, Alabama, devoted to the care and training of people with disabilities. These films—designated as the "Multi-handicapped Series"—have received much less attention than Wiseman's earlier work, as if films about disability mark a drastic departure from his previous award-winning productions, such as *Titicut Follies* (1967) and *Hospital* (1970). The Multi-handicapped Series takes up general categories of disabled populations as discrete documentary topics: *Deaf, Blind, Multi-handicapped*, and *Adjustment and Work* (1986–87). His earlier films focus on a particular place: Titicut is the name of the psychiatric institution and "Hospital" indicates a particular medical edifice and its inhabitants. The latter series of films identify social and interpersonal structures developed in the name of specific conditions. Consequently, these films focus on the activities of professionals and practitioners in education, administration, and therapy, as well as the institutional roles designed for bodies marked as severely disabled.

The last two films of the series, *Adjustment and Work* and *Multi-handicapped*, express the insufficiencies of the earlier ones; rather than specifying a single impairment-based classification, the films take up a taxonomy of the multiple. "Multi-handicapped" is thus not only a clean-up category for bodies that do not fit exclusively into the first films, it indicates the overlapping and cross-disability excesses that all bodies present for medical and administrative taxonomists alike.

Disability theorists have yet to give sufficient attention to the history of cross-referential factors in labeling disabilities. An examination of eugenics in the United States and Europe in the early twentieth century shows, for instance, that while its proponents professed to target "the feebleminded," and while historians may simply assume that "feebleminded" indicates a range of people with cognitive and learning disabilities, the actual populations en-snared in the rubric manifested a sweeping range of anatomies.[2]

Yet, in contrast to its predecessor classification of "feebleminded," even to-day's category of "disability" does not effectively address the diagnostic cross-referencing of the multiple anomalies that partition disabled bodies into iso-late congregations. In the United States in the late twentieth century, the policy answer to feeblemindedness was a division of disabilities into a binary structure of orthopedic or cognitive. Such a development has left many lim-ited and cross-over bodies in a diagnostic no-body's land (although Foucault might appreciate this interstitial location as offering up some potential for mobility). To analyze this history, one needs to recognize the formation of today's disability category as an effect of new diagnostic regimes of power. It is a form of domination based upon the application of particularized diag-nostic pathologies that provide the basis for cordoning off bodies which fail to fit neatly within the cognitive/orthopedic binary. This new landscape of disability informs our analysis of contemporary institutionalization in Wise-man's documentary series.

NORTH AMERICAN INSTITUTIONAL CONTEXTS In his essay "The Politics of Health in the Eighteenth Century" (2000a), Foucault theorizes the removal of social deviants into institutions in the late eighteenth and early nineteenth centuries on very different political grounds. For Foucault, the acceptability of the institutional erasure of objectionable bodies primar-ily resulted from a collusion between state and medical authorities to purge the body politic: "The eighteenth-century problematization of noso-politics correlates not with a uniform trend of state intervention in the practice of medicine but, rather, with the emergence at a multitude of sites in the so-cial body of health and disease as problems requiring some form or other of collective control measures. Rather than being the product of a vertical initiative coming from above, noso-politics in the eighteenth century figures as a problem with a number of different origins and orientations, being the problem of the health of all as a priority for all, the state of health of a popu-lation as a general objective of policy" (92).

Although Foucault primarily addresses a Western European context, his arguments about national projects of purification prove applicable to early nineteenth-century North America. His institutional histories all culminate in an explanation of eugenics as the logical, and most violent, extension of modern technologies of power: "The body no longer has to be marked; it must be trained and re-trained; its time must be measured out and fully used;

its forces must be continually applied to labor" (2000b, 35). Foucault's analyses leave us at the threshold of eugenics, and the sweeping taxonomy of a subnormal class deemed feebleminded. The ministrations to a presumably proliferating class of defectives in the eugenics era gave birth to our own contemporary strategies of exclusion and annexation of disability populations.

As for histories of North American institutions, David J. Rothman (1971) offers an account of a dramatic proliferation of incarcerating setups that indicate a shift in attitudes and expectations about human differences. Rather than pursue the economic relations of charity set out by early European settlers, according to which incapacitated individuals were cared for within their own homes or the houses of neighbors, institutionalization transformed a communal obligation into an increasingly state-sponsored, and ultimately federal, practice. Rothman contends that such a turn can be understood, in part, by the early European immigrants' view of disability, and the poverty that it often spawned, as a natural feature of experience: "they [the colonials] saw no prospect of eliminating deviancy from their midst" (1971, 15). Prerevolutionary U.S. culture incorporated physical and cognitive differences into an overarching philosophy of humanity as inherently fragile and subject to varieties of physical and spiritual corruption. While asylum historians tend to overly romanticize these features of colonial attitudes toward kinds of disability, they do show a stark contrast to the rise of institutional incarceration in the nineteenth century.

For example, colonial Americans refrained from using prolonged incarceration as a solution to social conflict, although the appearance of mutant children or madness was often disastrously interpreted within a religious framework of satanic design.[3] The most common forms of punishment were bodily markings, such as clipping the ears or applying tongue sticks; banishment from the settlement; and in extreme cases, as during the witchcraft trials, hanging. Each of these social solutions borrowed from the corporeal practices at work in previous eras, when bodies were targeted in a visceral way. With the exception of those who were hanged (approximately twenty-nine middle-aged women from 1629 to 1689), the implementation of corporal strategies proved temporary and minimally invasive. Punishments had a specified duration, such as time in the stocks. Restriction of movement was limited in the sense that those found guilty could not return to their community. Incapacity and poverty were not punishable crimes, and the expectation was that families and communities would care for their own members.

Histories of American institutionalization explain subsequent changes as the result of a shift in this public ethos of charity. The professional consolidation of medicine, therapeutic sciences, and psychiatry secured the perpetuation of institutions that would soon be designated as key sites for social engineering efforts. Physical and cognitive differences lost their status as inevitable, natural biological phenomena and became targets for medical intervention. The deviant body became a blight to be eradicated and an anomaly to be actively corrected through the use of increasingly invasive treatment programs.

At first, institutions had operated upon the premise that disabled bodies could be more adequately cared for within professional structures: extradition from public life for a brief period of time, combined with medical cures and immersion in nature, would ultimately result in social reintegration.[4] By 1830, a mere ten years after the initial establishment of many asylums in the United States, rehabilitation goals were recognized as a sham by medical and administrative professionals. As a consequence, with little planning the institutions devolved into permanent custodial facilities. The violent paradox of this development resides in the notion that ten years of institutional erasure provided a public with an appreciation for the removal of deviance that it would never relinquish.

COMPLIANT BODIES To comprehend institutions from the inside, one must turn away from external historical accounts of architecture and institutions, and toward Foucault's history of subjection. Across his institutional histories is an informing premise that surveillance comes to gradually supplant the corporeal model of punishment developed in the Middle Ages. To chart this transformation of the punitive mechanisms implemented by the state, Foucault also traces out the relationship of regimes of control over the body as an inherently plastic medium, one that can be made to speak the "truth" of an otherwise intangible moral core. In other words, the body becomes a locus for manipulation of social authority, both political and professional. Throughout his career, Foucault maintained a consistent view: power appears by virtue of its ability to make the body display, as if symptomatic and tangible, an internal disorder. Bodies provide the medium upon which, in the phrasing of Elaine Scarry (1985), the hidden interior becomes manifest upon the surface of the world.[5]

In a corporeal regime, the body must be made to bear witness to an otherwise internal deviance. The Middle Ages gave birth to corporeal coercion, whereby behavior was regulated through the infliction of pain and/or visible marks upon the external body. Backs are scarred by whips to punish waywardness; hands or fingers are amputated to punish thievery; the socially "sick" are forced to adorn their clothing with symbols that announce their transgressions, such as adultery or racial impurity. Corporeal discipline aims to bring the body into compliance with its "secret" truth by marking the exterior in some discernible manner. This kind of discipline is essentially a discursive order grafted upon the body in order to visually articulate morals and laws.

The flip side of the corporeal strategy is an overreliance on readings of the symbology of the body. While the unmarked or undermarked body must be made to physically manifest the signs of behavioral impropriety, the discernibly deviant body played host to fantasies of criminality and signatures of the supernatural. For instance, in the late 1500s Michel de Montaigne argued that French jails were filled with cripples and the mad who had been accused of witchcraft and other socially defined immoralities (1971a, 790). Different bodies marked as deviant are always at risk in historical moments when physiognomic principles reign supreme. One could argue that, since the Enlightenment, physiognomy has gone underground only to resurface in the scientific guise of empirical practices. Modern diagnostic taxonomies, from dermatology to genetic mutations, continue to orchestrate visible signs into empirical classifications of extraordinarily diverse phenomenon.

In the burgeoning network of institutions during the 1820s that included almshouses, workhouses, asylums, and hospitals, the bodies of those deemed crippled, lame, sickly, mad, and impoverished were incarcerated at alarming rates. In the United States, the period 1820–60 saw the escalation of incarcerated subjects in asylums alone go from hundreds to twenty thousand bodies (Rothman 1971, 209). Foucault argues that the panoptic era approached "the 'subject' stricken with illness" as disqualified or "stripped of any power and any knowledge concerning his illness" (1997, 49). The nineteenth-century asylum system, in particular, sought to eradicate the participation of the incarcerated as its primary mission in order to augment and solidify the authority of psychiatrists, doctors, and rehabilitation administrators wielding the power of diagnosis and human research design. As a result of the discounting of any input from the incarcerated themselves, the power of classification and treatment regimes became the exclusive property of various professions seeking to define expertise and thus secure cultural autonomy.

FILM METHODS AND TRAINING METHODOLOGIES   Wiseman provides a visual theory of contemporary institutional training and work that parallels the insidious reforms to penal history that Foucault theorizes, in *Madness and Civilization* (1988b), as a matter of false liberation. While Foucault's work traced a spread of disciplinary practices from the recesses of asylums and workhouses into every cranny of social existence, Wiseman's films return to the institution to assess the state of confinement practices today. By allowing the camera to linger on the banal details of the day-to-day time-management procedures of institutional work and school-day existence, Wiseman shows how institutions, by their nature, coerce acceptable behaviors and restrict bodily movements as their primary tactic. The façade of forced incarceration has dramatically transformed into a seemingly benign mimicry of a bourgeois existence beyond the walls of the institution.

This institutional process at first strikes the viewer as fairly minimal. Unlike the programs of their predecessor institutions that proliferated in Europe and America during the nineteenth century, the modern-day programs in Wiseman's films take place in structures where the residents move relatively freely through labyrinthine hallways of painted cinder block into classroom-like cul-de-sacs where they receive instruction.

Wiseman's films take singular local examples only to provide the vantage point of a vast social overview; in other words, by mining a specific institutional site, the filmmaker allows the viewer to gain a sense of contemporary North American institutionalization practices in general. However, in turning the (camera) gaze upon the (professional) gazers, Wiseman's reversals can often further efface those subject to professional scrutiny. In the Multi-handicapped Series the gazed-upon include the clients, confined, patients, or "subjugated subjectivities." Subjugated subjectivities may be made interchangeable with the Marxist notion of subproletariat, a term that fits well in the case of Wiseman's Multi-handicapped Series. After all, products of industries for the handicapped have historically been designated as a matter of therapy, not *work*. Subproletariat labor represents work efforts that redound to an institutional design, and not to an individual or laborer's creative efforts. The silencing locations, the places that muffle voices, impede narrative, and disrupt the individuation of memoirs and recollections, challenge the client's sense of things *within* institutional sites. To sustain this authority, institutional clinical practices ensure that practitioners refute, verify, or qualify all client-subjects' expressions as patient claims rather than clinical knowledge.

Wiseman's ethnographic tactics leave the perception that institutional exposés will yield little in the way of direct disability perspectives. Though we never hear voices responding to the filmmaker's direct inquiry, and we rarely observe direct eye-contact appeals to viewer involvement, we eavesdrop on professional modes and best-practices utterances from professionals and clients enacting and reiterating professional and rhetorical strictures. In this way, audiences seeking out disability perspectives view the predicament and management of disabled subjects. They witness the participatory power-grid that restricts rhetorical possibilities and what Ross Chambers (1991) calls "room to maneuver" within systems. It is this metastructural critique of institutional operations in the Multi-handicapped Series films that most closely mirrors Foucault's analytical methods: the experiences of the interned are eclipsed by the grander narrative of power and its operations.

Like Foucault's selection of the celebrated nineteenth-century institutional reformers, Samuel Tukes and Pinel, as central figures in *Madness and Civilization*, Wiseman only films at locations known for their progressive, humanistic standards. In tandem with Foucault, Wiseman limits his recording to exemplary professional sites and scenarios: open curricula, well-funded schools, painstaking teachers, well-meaning administrators. Each cultural critic serves up locations celebrated for their development of humane methods.[6]

Institutional subalterns in Wiseman's films respond to professional query and routine. But the issue of silencing remains profound, with interaction occurring under guided spaces and professions directed to run interference on private or cross-inmate discourse. At institutional sites where labor is not recognized as labor, where residents are thus not proletariat but subproletariat, where voting rights are in contention, and where voices are only reasonable when responsive and recognizable within disciplinary, professional, and rehabilitative frameworks, we are reminded that colonization, work colonies, work camps, or sheltered workshops remain common practices with respect to contemporary disabled populations.

Residents remain unintelligible in their very availability to endless analysis, not just routine surveillance, but membership in research pools that are made to release evidence for disciplinary and professional knowledge. The presence of the helping sciences—therapists, employment specialists, and social workers—is responsible for the narrative of today's humane institution. In other words, even though institutional locations may deny nearly every basic human right, they continue to count as socially acceptable solutions.

In a Foucauldian vein, Wiseman's camera seeks to allow contradictory practices to trace out their own self-justifications—eventually implicating themselves. The nearly invisible editing effort is constructed in such a way that institutions need no outside exposure of their disastrous potential. Instead, the portrayal of the banality of institutional life provides the context for a viewing experience that leaves a distasteful residue behind—as if we were privy to a voyeuristic episode that stains us with a knowledge we might rather not possess.

Wiseman's first film, *Titicut Follies*, was banned for nearly thirty years in Massachusetts on the basis that the filmmaker had violated incarcerated inmates' privacy. Yet what strikes viewers of Wiseman's oeuvre is how few examples there are of objectifying film methods. In interviews Wiseman famously responds that the Titicut institution itself, and not his film, engaged in systemic violations of privacy. What is uncomfortable in Wiseman's documentaries is not our experience of an invasive camera that bores into the humiliating private experiences of those who have no choice. Rather, we squirm at how our institutions ultimately rob people of the trappings of privacy to which we have become so accustomed as middle-class citizens. In other words, Wiseman's films transgress upon the intimate lives of incarcerated individuals in order to expose justifications for institutional denials of privacy.

BLIND CANE TRAVEL   A common visual theme in the Multi-handicapped Series is that of cane travel training for individuals who have become blind. *Multi-handicapped*, *Adjustment and Work*, and *Blind* all begin with scenes of blind cane travel training. Wiseman's analysis of disciplinary tactics begins in this encounter with therapeutic techniques. For instance in *Multi-handicapped* a bus pulls up to a suburban sidewalk, the doors open, and two individuals disembark—the sighted instructor/bus driver and the blind student. As the camera follows their activities in a medium shot, we are made privy to the ways in which one is trained to be blind (visually impaired individuals often share the joke that they "have to go learn how to be blind today"). The audience and the newly blind student take up a counter-relationship to each other with respect to a sighted hierarchy that is commonplace in contemporary culture: the audience watches as the instructor looks on silently in order to observe and evaluate the proficiency of the blind cane traveler in the techniques of caning.

This process of "learning to be blind" involves more than just the effective manipulation of a prosthetic instrument. A dual form of discipline is at work in these scenes, in which the student learns to maneuver a cane while also being subject to the evaluative oversight of the instructor. The audience is expected to do little more than take up an already extant objectifying position with respect to the blind individual's mobilization of him- or herself in the world. There is nothing new to this relationship, and the scenes quickly grow wearisome unless we undertake an analysis of our own familiarity with an objectifying stare. The subject of cane travel evaluation not only undergoes a surveillance of technique and entry into an idea of independence founded upon conformity to the sighted world's conventions of mobility, but also, and perhaps more important, becomes the object of a discomforting observational scrutiny.

The new cane traveler is exported into the space of the suburbs in the way one would bring a new teenage driver to an empty parking lot. The practice of operating a motorized vehicle and the trained arc of a cane delivers one into a ritual of initiation: both operations are performed in the name of "breaking one in" to the discipline of a prostheticized existence. The body becomes an extension—in Marshall McLuhan's sense (1964)—of the device rather than the other way around. The sighted cane travel overseer also becomes an artificial appendage to the sight-impaired. The relationship of power and dependency enacted in the process of cane tutoring does not diminish with the cane traveler's extrication from the relationship of tutelage: an evaluative gaze is internalized as a key component of walking itself.

Thus, newly blind subjects learn to walk with canes while their sighted instructors badger them to make exaggerated arcs with their canes—that is, arcs that move from one side of the sidewalk to the other—an impractical technique to use on sidewalks that are occupied by others. The exaggerated arc that the cane makes not only extends one's capacity to be mobile in a sighted world but also continuously marks one as noticeably deviant. Even after the instructor removes him- or herself from the scene of instruction, the cane traveler continues to carry an internalized version of an evaluating gaze. In short, the technique of cane traveling comes with the initiation of a visually impaired individual into a panoptic scheme that follows her wherever she goes. Conditioned to being watched as the primary experience of visual impairment, a blind cane user experiences life constructed as a gaze that cannot see back.

NAPKIN FOLDING AND OTHER USEFUL INSTITUTIONAL SKILLS The irony of institutional relationships (such as the one inaugurated during cane travel instruction) is the degree to which the helping practices of training and rehabilitation come to be associated with objectification and the subtleties of social subjugation. This dual structure of assistance and objectification permeates the institutional settings into which Wiseman's cameras bring us. As we move from cane training episodes to the classrooms of the Helen Keller Institute for the Deaf and Blind, we encounter an odd

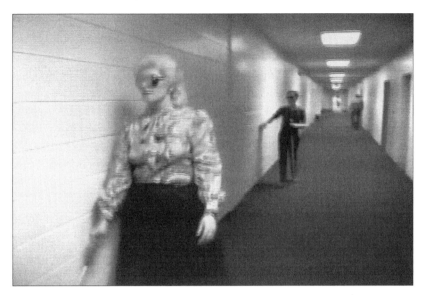

BLIND CANE TRAVELERS AT TRAINING SCHOOL, FROM FREDERICK WISEMAN'S FILM
«WORK AND ADJUSTMENT» (1986)

aporia. All of the administrators and teachers of the Alabama institution participate in the production of rhetoric about returning its residents to the community, yet they pursue practices that prepare the residents for little more
than a future within the sheltered society of the institution. As one adminis-
trator explains to a group of nondisabled workers, the institute seeks to train
residents "to function in an open or *sheltered* society." The positioning of the
connective *or* in this comment demonstrates the conflict that undergirds all
institutional objectives. Even in the rhetoric of "return to society," custodial
institutions struggle to hold onto their residents as a function of their own
livelihood. The training of docile subjects within institutions takes a great
deal of time and an extraordinary amount of energy. This investment of resources makes the creation of good (read: "docile") institutional subjects the
primary unacknowledged aim of institution staff.

Release into the community of the successfully trained institutional subject is difficult for several reasons. First, the institution's mission is premised
upon its own internalization of prejudicial beliefs about those who make
up its population. Second, a disciplined subject is the most valuable of all
commodities in an institution whose structure struggles to retain a hold on
those in whom it has invested its resources. Third, the disciplined subject

147

has been prepared to lead a life of institutionalization, not one of independence. Preparation, in the regulated life of institutions, does not prepare one for successful navigation of the outside world, for the structured regimen of institutional organization infiltrates the fibers of one's being. Thus, subjects become increasingly adapted to living a life whose parameters are no larger than the institutional grounds.

We never witness anyone's reintegration into a larger society in any of the four films that make up Wiseman's Multi-handicapped Series. Instead, we watch inmates navigate a structure that seems to fold in upon itself. Classrooms are buried within a labyrinthine organization whose recesses seem opposed to interaction with the outside world. Like the institution itself, Wiseman's films prevent the viewer from obtaining a relational vantage point to the larger world. Hallways and rooms of nondescript cinder block provide a minimalist setting for institutional activities. The lack of windows in any of the rooms seals inmates within an insulated environment. We follow residents through the structure; rarely, however, does the camera take us outside the compound.

On the rare occasions when we do exit the compound, we witness a structured and interlocked series of awnings and sidewalks that channel residents from one building to the next as if the concrete routes are determined and invariable. The variegated bodies that traverse this network situate themselves in stark contrast to the uniform aesthetic of the institution itself. One might easily conclude that the institution's organization and logic are primarily intended to diminish or even thwart the diversity of those who inhabit it. The uniformity of the institution's operations demands a conformity that is commensurate with the banal setting of the edifice itself.

In one film of the series, we witness team meeting participants discussing the case of a resident who will not sleep enough hours during the night. This practice of "not sleeping enough" is said to make the resident insufficiently obedient for institutional training during the day. Her disruptions and resistance to practicing the regimen of training mark her for further intervention: not a change in her program of study, but an increase in the level of medication administered to her at night. Indeed, the institution resists all efforts to flout its rituals of participation. Medication serves as a key weapon in its arsenal of coercion. As the girl's teacher explains near the end of the meeting: "I know it's going to be hard, but you know—this sleeping—I'm just afraid that it's going to take her down and get her sick . . . and we can't have that—being sick." The issue in such exchanges is not indifference or disregard on the part of the institution's staff. On the contrary, the rigidity of the institution's governmental rationale dictates that all staff exercise only limited options for action with respect to the treatment that they accord residents.

In a later scene, we witness the sleepless girl in question, Cheryl, performing her training regimen beside her teacher. This training, which consists of rote repetitions of sorting yellow pegs into the holes that have been made in a plastic board, provides a window into the monotony of institutional life. The teacher urges, encourages, and disciplines her student's willingness to sort the pegs into the allotted holes over and over again. The monotonous nature of the task provides the viewer with an understanding of institutional objectives: occupy residents with a series of operations that add up to little more than a future of continuous institutionalization. The goal of even low-level vocational education becomes a farce at this point. One must *do* something to fill up an institutional day, whose major objective transforms into an effort to keep its residents out of trouble and busy. As Wiseman's films demonstrate with painstaking observational techniques (and in the painfully plodding nature of his ethnographic process), one's time-in is ultimately defined by the extent to which an inmate successfully adjusts to the monotony of an absolutely structured life.

The significance of the film's location in the Helen Keller Institute comes into full relief when the object of the training shifts from the pegboard activity to facecloth folding. Wiseman depicts the instruction, and the attention that the teacher gives to it, in a manner that recalls a famous scene in *The Miracle Worker* (1962): Annie Sullivan (Anne Bancroft) announces with excitement that Helen (Patty Duke) has successfully folded her napkin for the first time. In exultation Helen's mother repeats, against a tumultuous sky, "Folded her napkin! She folded her napkin!" In the institutional enactment of this sentimental and civil goal, the teacher enthusiastically kisses and hugs her deaf-blind pupil when she has performed the specified maneuvers that achieve the desired end (a folded facecloth).

By contrast, the deaf-blind girl in Wiseman's film appears to display utter indifference to the practice. We witness her withdrawing from the activity and recoiling from the affectionate reactions of the teacher. When the teacher reprimands her pupil for failing to make a clean edge, the girl makes evident that she regards the procedure as one that demands a degree of attention that the specified goal (facecloth folding) does not deserve. As we see throughout the film, however, the teachers and administrators of the institute discount this point of view because they have already precluded recognition that their pupils possess the subjectivities that would make it possible to enjoy or dislike the tasks to which they are assigned. Put directly, the film

Multi-handicapped demonstrates the degree to which this deaf-blind student has been transformed into the automaton that the institution staff assumes her to be.

Through the repetition of folding a washcloth, one acquires a series of necessary institutional skills: first, practicing a domesticated version of independence that allows the overseers and instructors of the institution more free time to pursue other objectives; second, overseeing the government of the self that Foucault has diagnosed as the key form of control practiced in Western societies; third, undertaking various activities as a tool of occupation during the regulation of time over the course of each institutional day; and fourth, performing the obedience expressed by the willingness to fold one's napkin over and over again as a viable skill.

In other words, the mythic napkin-folding scene of *The Miracle Worker* is transubstantiated into an allegory of the promised entrance into a future integrated life. Yet the activity itself bears no relation to that illusory goal. Instead, it provides the institution with a model that superficially mimics the values of middle-class existence. While few of the residents of the institution will go on to realize the elusive goal of integration, the institution seeks to engage all of its residents in a performance of appearances that lend a middle-class respectability to them. Just as in Foucault's critique of Tukes's domesticating model, the institution becomes the simulacrum of middle-class domesticity in a way that entrenches those values on the outside as natural.

The message that comes across most poignantly in Wiseman's films is that something more subtle than violence against bodies characterizes modern institutions: namely, the regimentation of time into minute segments of trivial occupation. As Foucault argues, this oversight of space and time distributes and compartmentalizes bodies into spaces that allow for optimum oversight and regulation: "Discipline . . . arranges a positive economy. It poses the principle of a theoretically ever-growing use of time: exhaustion rather than use; it is a question of extracting, from time, ever more available moments and, from each moment, ever more useful forces" (1995, 154). The point of successful napkin folding is less the achievement of a desirable skill than the entrance into an apparatus of power that conditions subjects by enthralling them to a microscopic domain of bodily instrumentation. One *folds* successfully not because the task is mastered but because the body is trained to perform rote actions in a sequence. One moves one's arms and hands to accomplish a task; however, the task itself is not completed so much as the maneuvers that lead to the completion of the task are fulfilled. As the girl's hands appear to hover over the folding operation in indecision, the

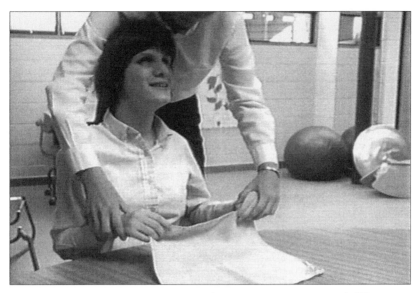

FACE-CLOTH FOLDING, FROM WISEMAN'S FILM «MULTI-HANDICAPPED» (1986)

teacher prompts her arm with a nudge to complete the activity. In this way, the teacher establishes a mechanism that proves merely functional and the pupil's body is placed in its service.

INDEPENDENCE IN ISOLATION Resistance to such regimentation and to its ultimate goal—the physical partitioning that dissuades, and indeed prevents, residents from engaging in intimacy and meaningful interaction with each other—is rarely on display in Wiseman's films. There are key moments when Wiseman's camera breaks through the institutional narrative into a scene of intimacy and significant communication, but they are few and far between. In one key moment in *Multi-handicapped*, a deaf-blind and deaf cross-racial pair communicate with hand/touch signing in a recreation room with a pool table. Another pointed episode in *Deaf* shows groups of inmates happily conversing with each other in a flurry of sign language exchanges. *Adjustment and Work* follows two blind students down a hallway as a more experienced blind woman helps a sight-impaired man understand the workings of the training in which they will both participate. These scenes prove singular moments that contrast starkly with the rest of the film's focus on institutional operations and administration.

Yet, the primary, and prevailing, objective of the series is to demonstrate the degree to which institutions prove successful in keeping apart inmates

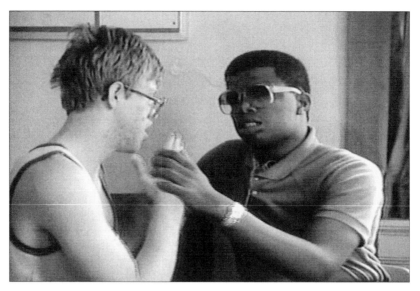

DEAF-BLIND COMMUNICATION IN POOL ROOM FROM WISEMAN'S FILM
«MULTI-HANDICAPPED» (1986)

who share a relatively small space. The extreme individuation and partitioning of the institution circulates as the goal of all institutional staff curriculum meetings. The point of institutional objectives is never to cultivate an
intimacy and interdependency among the residents that might make institutional life habitable for those who are most in need of the comfort that
comes from communal interdependence. Instead, the tasks of the contemporary institution are particular and individual. Isolation is not accomplished
by confining subjects in a cell, but rather by maintaining what one adminis-
trator calls a "flexible and individualized program of study." Residents pursue
self-care and vocational training as an ironic expression of the institution's
efforts to help them achieve independence. What results from engaging in
these practices of self-care is extreme compartmentalization and distance
from one's fellow inmates.

In the Multi-handicapped Series, independence is slowly transformed
into its antithesis: realization of institutional dependency that results from
a lack of contact with one's peers, relatives, and society in general. In the
institution, instruction functions on a vertical axis of power from adminis-
trator to teacher, from teacher to student; rarely does educational practice
occur there on a horizontal axis of shared endeavor and friendship. For instance, in the film *Adjustment and Work* Wiseman presents a series of shel-

tered workshop arrangements where residents labor six days a week for scant pay. Each worker is caught on film occupying his or her own niche in the institutional mechanism. Sewers work their machines without repartee with their fellow sewers; stampers monotonously turn out labels for clothing; belt-makers buckle and rebuckle their products for packaging in absolute silence; backpack straps are hoisted onto singular hooks and excess string is cut off with a small scissor in absolute silence. Only the whir of machinery can be heard in the background. In scenes of profound alienation, the workers are cut off from each other until the shift ends and the buzzer sounds. In each scenario, the production floor is filled with the sounds of machinery that has entirely displaced the conversation of workers.

The individualized training tasks that are introduced to younger children at the institution lead directly to their realization in a modern sweatshop. When one watches all four of the films in the Multi-handicapped Series, one can see how Wiseman has connected the two different training orders—vocational school and sweatshop—into one apparatus. As elementary students place pegs in form-boards, their adult counterparts zip and buckle and snap in a series of parallel, perfunctory operations. Each worker becomes a cog in the industrial wheel of the institution, and education becomes a foundational step toward fulfilling one's future place in the labor assembly line. As Foucault might put it, "this is a functional reduction of the body. But it is also an insertion of this body-segment in a whole ensemble over which it is articulated" (1995, 164).

Beyond the controlled labor practices, Wiseman's portrayals emphasize that the institution dedicates itself most fiercely to a regulation of sexuality. Because sexuality, in its broadest sense, connotes a site of interaction unregulated by states and institutions, the segregation of bodies lurks as the ultimate institutional prerogative. Like its eugenics-era predecessors, institutions for the feebleminded, the institution of Wiseman's films targets sexuality as its foremost object of obsessive intervention. As the institutional director in *Deaf* makes clear in a meeting with his employees, regulation of sexuality is their responsibility not only when they are on the job but even when they are off the job. He instructs his employees, "If for any reason you happen to be around campus [knowing, titillated laughter arises from the staff] in the evenings, it would be very much appreciated if you would drive through the campus and if you see something that's not correct, stop and talk with them [the inmates and dorm parents] about it." To underscore this point, the director tells a story about his discovery of residents necking one night on the unlit patio of Grace Hall. In these scenarios, abstinence functions as coerced control of sexuality—a goal that is tacitly understood among administrators, teachers, and employees.

In the concluding night scenes in both *Adjustment and Work* and *Blind*, we witness the residents methodically being put to bed. Just as workshops and training classes segregate students in disparate areas of the production floor or classrooms, the night rituals that surround bedtime in the institution are meant to prevent unwanted physical contact among its residents. Evenings are orchestrated with an eye toward separating residents to the greatest degree possible. Even in the relatively close space of residence halls, the inmates find themselves quickly separated from each other after nightfall and sequestered within their own designated bedrooms. This is the one time that physical isolation is architecturally sanctioned.

The pursuit of this subtle, yet pervasive, effort to cordon off inmates from meaningful contact with each other within the social *and* individual spaces of institutions functions as the cornerstone of institutional structures. Control is evident not in physical threat or in the rhetorical abuse of its inmate populations (as was evident in *Titicut Follies*), but rather in an orchestrated logic of isolation within a teeming social space. Each part of the day is saturated with techniques of individuation. In Foucault's words:

> This machinery works space in a much more flexible and detailed way. It does this first of all on the principle of elementary location or *partitioning*. Each individual has his own place; and each place its individual. Avoid distributions in groups; break up collective dispositions; analyze confused massive or transient pluralities. Disciplinary space tends to be divided into as many sections as there are bodies or elements to be distributed. One must eliminate the effects of imprecise distributions, the uncontrolled disappearance of individuals, their diffuse circulation, their unstable and dangerous coagulation; it was a tactic of anti-desertion, anti-vagabondage, anti-concentration. Its aim was to establish presences and absences, to know where and how to locate individuals, to set up useful communications, to interrupt others, to be able at each moment to supervise the conduct of each individual, to assess it, to judge it, to calculate its qualities or merits. (1995, 143; original emphasis)

Disciplinary space is fully recognizable in Wiseman's visual anthropology of today's disability institutions. Documenting the observational stare of the cane travel instructor, the disciplinary tutoring sessions received by blind workers, the employability meetings that assess an individual's work history and physical and moral character, and curriculum meetings that rate disabilities into levels of "trainability," the Multi-handicapped Series illuminates the operations of contemporary *discipline* as that which "organizes an analytical space" (1995, 143).

Like the institutional subjects they treat, the Multi-handicapped Series films reflect deep-seated discomfort with the topic of disability and our society's efforts to relegate those who occupy the category to invisibility. Institutionalization is the adoption of a management scheme that seeks to solve the social dilemmas of disability—physical and intellectual access, functional variations, aesthetic differences, pathologized states of embodiment, the potent knowledge of the rejected—through a literal removal of the source of the conflict. Yet this approach to the subject reproduces the conflict itself from one generation to the next by re-creating human differences into mysteries. How do we reacquaint ourselves with those marked as deviant while banishing them from social view? Such practices replicate foundational eugenics tactics in our own contemporary moment. Wiseman's films prompt us to interrogate our cultural investment in cultural locations of disability that do not share the stage of the social as a most basic human right.

FIVE

Body Genres and Disability Sensations | *The Challenge of the New Disability Documentary Cinema*

SPECTACULAR DISABILITIES One of the more memorable scenes from Robert Zemeckis's *Forrest Gump* (1994) shows the double-amputee war veteran, Lieutenant Dan, lifting himself from a seated position on the floor up into his wheelchair. The scene is pointed for a variety of reasons. Most obviously, moving one's body from the floor to a wheelchair solely with one's arms is a feat of strength and skill. Further, the scene provides the viewer with a unique opportunity to stare at the dynamics of a physical transition we rarely witness—particularly from the safe perspective offered by a movie theater seat (or one's own furniture). Finally, a viewer's knowledge that the actor, Gary Sinise, is able-bodied encourages him or her to marvel at the special effects required to simulate amputation.

The identification of the latter two layers, imaginative involvement and spectatorial pleasure, involved in performances of disability supplies an unanalyzed nexus of viewer identification—or dis-identification, as the case may be. As a witness to this spectacle the viewer is offered a unique opportunity, since the physical prowess involved is rivaled only by the technological wizardry of erasing the actual legs of an able-bodied actor.

156

Special effects threaten to overwhelm the more tried-and-true filmic spectacle of a disabled body navigating an environment in its own unique manner.

To interrogate this nexus between spectator and the filmed disabled body
as a spectacle, we must inevitably delve into the psychic structures that give
meaning to disability as a constructed social space. This space of psychic
interaction does not exist universally, but a limited theoretical foray into this
well-traversed arena of film criticism should provide opportunities heretofore unrecognized in disability studies.[1] In mainstream fiction film—defined
for our purposes as U.S.-based productions organized around principles of
continuity editing associated with the Hollywood film industry—disability
supplies an important opportunity to feed two seemingly antithetical modes
of visual consumption: the desire to witness body-based spectacles and a
desire to know an object "empirically" as an aftereffect of viewing. While
mainstream fiction film productions have been exclusively associated with
the first viewing position—entertainment through the witness of spectacle—
film technology's long historical relationship with the scientific gaze also
needs to be theorized.

Throughout the nineteenth and twentieth centuries, what we have called
cultural locations of disability were produced primarily through the scrutiny
of disabled bodies as research objects in the investigations of medicine, rehabilitation, and other fields devoted primarily to empiricisms of the body.
Film spectatorship borrows from these weighty disciplinary practices in that
bodies marked as anomalous are offered for consumption as objects of necessary scrutiny—even downright prurient curiosity. As Elizabeth Cowie (1999)
says of documentary film, "In curiosity, the desire to see is allied with the
desire to know through seeing *what cannot normally be seen*, that is, what is
normally veiled or hidden from sight" (28; emphasis added). Disability plays
this primary role in most Hollywood film productions, by allowing viewers
to witness spectacles of bodily difference without fear of recrimination by the
object of this gaze. Social conventions of normalcy as products of historical
viewing practices are highlighted in mainstream film representations of disability by the cultivation of a belief that one is witnessing a previously secret
or hidden phenomenon.

Cowie's repetition of the word *normally* provides a key to theorizing film
spectator relationships to the screening of disabled bodies. To a significant
degree, film produces interest in its objects through the promise of providing bodily differences as an exotic spectacle. What can "normally be seen" or
"what is normally veiled or hidden from sight" secures a privileged position
for disabled bodies on film because they promise an opportunity to practice a

form of objectifying ethnography. That which is created as off-limits in public spaces garners the capital of the unfamiliar. Film promotes its status as a desirable cultural product partly through its willingness to recirculate bodies typically concealed from view. In this way, the closeting of disabled people from public observation exacts a double marginality: *disability extracts one from participation while also turning that palpable absence into the terms of one's exoticism*. Film spectators arrive at the screen prepared to glimpse the extraordinary body displayed for moments of uninterrupted visual access—a practice shared by clinical assessment rituals associated with the medical gaze. Consequently, the "normative" viewing instance is conceived as that which is readily available for observation in culture. To a great extent, film's seduction hinges on securing audience interest through the address of that which is constructed as "outside" a common visual field.

In this chapter we set out some critical modes of spectatorship generated by conventions of disability portrayal in film. This is not an exhaustive effort by any means, nor do we intend to imply that these are the only viewing positions available. Rather we aim to identify some significant viewing relationships commonly cultivated in mainstream film. Visual media analysis in disability studies has made some initial efforts to critique filmic portrayals of disability as predominantly negative and stereotypical, yet in focusing interest exclusively in this area, little attention has been paid to the dynamic relationship between viewers and disabled characters.[2] Since, as we have argued, most people make the majority of their life acquaintances with disabled people in film, television, and literature, the representational milieu of disability provides a critical arena for disability studies analysis (Mitchell and Snyder 2000, 52). The analysis of film images of disability provides an opportune location of critical intervention, a form of discursive rehab upon the site of our deepest psychic structures mediating our reception of human differences.

EXCESSIVE FILM BODIES To a significant extent this chapter owes a debt to the work of feminist film critic Linda Williams. Williams has followed up feminism's efforts to anatomize the complex space that exists between images and their spectatorial reception by audience members. In particular, Williams concentrates—following on work by film theorist Teresa De Lauretis (1984)—on women as imbibers of their own filmed images. While De Lauretis theorized this psychic structure as the site of a "double pleasure" where women identify both with the masochistic objectification of female characters and the sadistic position of the prototypical masculine viewer to whom film is often addressed, Williams probes a variety of genres and thus, a variety of potential modes of viewer identification. In essence, Williams's analyses fracture the act of viewing into a rich multiplicity of visual relations based on cross-genre comparison—particularly with respect to films she identifies as existing to elicit extreme bodily sensations in audiences. This attention to cross-genre structures of audience identification allows Williams to de-universalize the more monolithic cast of De Lauretis's influential analysis. We will briefly review Williams's arguments as a predecessor text to our own deliberations. Williams's film bodies provide a key entry into our own speculations about the imagery of disability in mainstream Hollywood visual texts.

In her essay "Film Bodies: Gender, Genre, and Excess" (1999), Williams opens by arguing that film bodies play at a critical nexus in film viewing practices. Rather than abstracting the body at a distance, "body genres" such as melodrama, horror, and pornography focus on the production of palpable sensation. Their filmic power depends upon the ability to situate the body in the throes of extreme sensation characterized by stimuli produced by pain, hysteria, terror, sobbing—in other words, those bodily sensations that might be characterized as excessive. This notion of the constitutive excess produced as the key commodity in body genres allows Williams to stipulate heightened somatic involvement as the goal of certain visual genres. In other words, films participating in the body genres target the visceral emotional life of the body both on screen and in viewing audiences. This analysis situates a phenomenological mode of spectatorship as a process critical to the interpretation of cinema and other visual media.

According to contemporary film criticism, a film's success depends upon its ability to generate sensations, as well as replicate successful formula plotlines. Hence, we can best understand films as *body genres* since, for example, melodrama, horror, and pornography are primarily experienced in terms of the spectacular moments that generate sensations in the bodies of their viewers (Williams 1999, 702). For example, in melodrama a character's loss overtakes audience members, who are encouraged to experience a similar sensation—usually toward another human being or a body function. In horror films the terror of an unexpected meeting with the villain (often disabled), and anxiety over potential or actual violence, produces an accord of sensations between characters and members of a viewing audience. In pornography, sexual arousal and orgasm performed by the film's characters are likewise intended to produce similar responses for the viewers. Each of these genre formulas depends upon its ability to cultivate an overidentification between viewer and imperiled character on screen to achieve its desired effects. The body is endangered as a staple plot element in these works, and the degree to which audiences identify with the impending loss of control in their own bodies will determine the ultimate "success" of the film. Body films attempt to situate the filmed body in the throes of excessive emotion as an object of mediation for an anticipated viewer's own experience of embodied peril.

Critics of such films often deem "inappropriate" what Williams defines as "an apparent lack of proper esthetic distance, a sense of over-involvement in sensation and emotion" (1999, 5). The viewer surfaces from such film experiences betrayed by a sense of manipulation; audience members find themselves immersed in the "violence" of emotional excess and experience the aftermath of such immersion as a "cheap thrill." One could analyze Williams's analysis as a theory of guilty pleasures in cinema. All of these generic forms depend on the portrayal of body spectacle to one degree or another: the horror movie provides violence as a visceral mechanism of terror; the melodrama uses pathos toward bodily loss as the primary tool to evoke intense grief or sadness; and the pornographic film involves the explicit portrayal of body functions usually ruled out of bounds by classical cinema. Each form of bodily display provides film viewers with an opportunity to "surrender" to extreme sensations rarely available in their daily lives.

Rather than follow certain feminist approaches that condemn such spectacles or see them as matters of "false consciousness" in female viewers who participate in their consumption, Williams contends that a multiplicity of viewing spaces exist within such products. In other words, rather than castigate such films for merely replicating the female viewer as "passive victim," she sees body genres as offering more than a simplistic formula of masochistic objectification. On the one hand, "identification is neither fixed nor entirely passive" (1999, 8); on the other, a viewer's oscillation among positions of power and passivity provides an opportunity to reconcile the *splintering* of self and other—at least for a while. Genre films set a field of signifiers into motion, and viewers try out various vantage points during the story. A pleasure of the multiple is at play in even the most hackneyed of formulas; therefore, Williams encourages a more complex examination of "the system and structure" of sensation (2).

Williams argues that by addressing historically persistent problems, such as sexuality, desire, and vulnerability, body genres provide a variety of "temporal structures [that] constitute the different utopian component of problem-solving in each form" (1999, 11). By taking up social issues that continue to resonate in the public context as "difficult," body genre films address the defining ambiguity of these problems through a perpetual recycling of their existence within the parameters of their plot structures. Thus, for Williams, the pleasure of horror results from its exposure of adolescent sexuality as not yet fully prepared for an encounter with a monster (as a symbol of insatiable sexual appetite); the investment in melodrama stems from a "quest for connection . . . tinged with the melancholy of loss" (ibid.); and in pornography one might characterize the dilemma as the coincidental encounter between "seducer and seduced" at just the right moment for the pursuit of mutual gratification. In each formula, timing becomes critical to the structural parameters of the genre. The screen bodies "suffer" at the hands of time when pursuits are defeated, deferred, or satiated. The popularity of these plots is based on their ability to dredge up longstanding social problems that expose viewers to irresolution as a "solution." Thus, the "resolution" comes about through the repetition of exposure to a social dilemma that can only be exposed rather than resolved.

To organize her thoughts on the operations at work in body genre films, Williams provides a diagram titled "An Anatomy of Film Bodies" that categorizes the mechanisms at work in each formula. Using bodily sensation as a tool for assessing each genre's operation, Williams anatomizes gendered responses. For our present purposes, the critical element of her diagram is the degree to which the sensations experienced by bodies on the screen and by the audience coincide. The ecstatic shudder evoked by the horror film, the tears produced by the melodrama, and the orgasm aroused by the pornographic all situate the body as seismic register of the genre film's successful application.

In her diagram, Williams maps out the gender of each genre's presumed target audience: melodrama appeals to girls and women, horror to adolescent boys, pornography to men. The diagram also identifies the prototypical affect associated with each formula from sadism (pornography) to sadomasochism (horror) to masochism (melodrama). In each case, the dominant production of the gendered viewer reinforces cultural scripts targeted at an audience's relationship to norms of gender and sexuality extant in Western narratives of heterosexuality.

Thus, Williams's "anatomy of film bodies" refuses simplistic dismissals of body genre films as crass or merely ideologically duplicitous, while using their fantasy structures as a means to expose ideologically invested formulas. As she explains, "body genres which may seem so violent and inimical to women cannot be dismissed as evidence of a monolithic or unchanging misogyny, as either pure sadism for male viewers or masochism for females" (1999, 12). Rather, body genres offer an entry into the complex structure of film fantasy within which we participate as members of a media culture.

If such a model can prove instructive for analyses of gendered pleasures and popular myths, we would argue a similar utility for explorations of disabled bodies as staple characterizations within these popular formulas. Williams's own analysis hits upon several conventions pertinent to disability in film without recognizing film's investment in what Elaine Scarry terms the "body in pain" (1985). In Williams's study, gender eclipses disability because she bypasses an analysis of the different body's pivotal function in the development of each genre.

Because body genres rely on extreme sensation, we argue that disability is as crucial as gender in the primal structuring fantasies of these formulas. Body genres are so dependent on disability as a representational device (a process we have referred to as "narrative prosthesis" [Mitchell and Snyder 2000, 6]) that each formula can be recognized by its reliance on particular kinds of disabled bodies to produce the desired sensational extremes. We recognize the "bumbling fool" of comedy (as in the screwball plots of the 1960s that featured later disability telethon sycophant Jerry Lewis), the disabled avenger of horror (as showcased in any number of psychological thrillers or monster plot formulas), or the long-suffering victim of melodrama, as in *Dark Victory* (1939), which starred Bette Davis as a young woman dying from some unspecified condition. Within such an analytical scheme we might also contemplate the various anatomical anomalies that drive pornography plots searching for the ultimate sexual encounter.

In every one of these cases we come upon a familiar body genre formula identified by Williams in her analysis of gender and sensation. Yet we can also identify representations of disability in each of these cinematic scenarios as a key form of embodiment that gives shape and structure to the formulas. Quite simply put: *disabled bodies have been constructed cinematically and socially to function as delivery vehicles in the transfer of extreme sensation to audiences.* Thus, an anatomy of disabled bodies can deepen our comprehension of the system and structure of body genres.

AN ANATOMY OF CINEMATIC DISABILITY While Williams's essay focuses primarily on the nature of sensations produced by body genres, a full analysis of their impact includes a discussion of the means by which such sensations are produced. This implies not just a theoretical analysis of psychic investments between characters and viewers, but also a scrutiny of the embodied conditions that play host to the generation of sensation in the first place. As a vehicle of sensation, disabled bodies play an important role as either the threatened producer of trauma (as in the case of the monstrous stalker) or as the threat toward the integrity of the able body (as in the case of the hereditary carrier of "defective" genes). The extreme sensations paralleled in screen bodies and audience responses rely, to a great extent, on shared cultural scripts of disability as that which must be warded off at all costs. Bodies are subjected to their worst fears of vulnerability and/or the already disabled body is scripted as out of control. The order and mastery associated with the nondisabled body often becomes the threat posed in these film formulas. This fantasy of bodily control among audience members becomes the target of body genres as a fiction deeply seated in the desire for an impossible dominion over our own capacities. At stake is what Foucault refers to as the government of the body, whereby individuals are produced as subjects responsible for policing their own bodily aesthetics, functions, and controls (2003, 48). In either case the disabled body in body genres surfaces as the locus of tension and the source of excessive sensation.

If productions of body genres display sensations that are, as Williams contends, on "the edge of respectable" (1999, 2), then one must contemplate the degree to which disabled bodies are made to demarcate the culturally policed borders of respectability itself. The designation of extreme sensations might be best characterized as a *response* to the "excesses" of human bodies displayed on the screen. In this manner we are not discussing a fact of bodies but rather a social investment in certain bodies' presumed proximity to abjectness. The "edge" implied by matters of respectability is that questions of social propriety always depend on something over which one has little to no control. A body of behaviors or actions deemed inappropriate depends on the degree to which one manages or masks the conditions of one's own materiality. Thus, in Tobin Siebers's (2004) terms, the disabled body is expected to engage in public "masquerades" of its own normalcy. "Success" in regard to disability (and all bodies in general) is judged according to one's ability to dissimulate actions or behaviors deemed aberrant and thus, unrespectable.

The "body genres" relate directly to the degree to which one commands the behaviors and capacities of one's own body. We know that such command is elusive at best, yet the "nonexcessive" body is defined by virtue of its ability to oversee and appropriately manage its own by-products. For instance, when the character played by John Belushi in *Animal House* (1978) performs the role of a human "zit" by stuffing his mouth with mashed potatoes and then violently ejecting the contents onto all around him, the scene produces a mixture of disgust and laughter that one equates with the essence of "gross" in comedy. The degree to which one experiences this reaction of disgust and laughter may be gendered in Williams's schema, but the vehicle of the sensation is a bodily function gone awry. The performance of a "zit" brings the question of such bodily operations into a public forum that is usually shielded from such unseemly subjects, while the characterization reveals a bodily "outburst" no longer under the complete dominion of a fully socialized body. Bodies must remain within certain boundaries, and their "leakage" beyond such parameters violates social expectations of propriety (the appropriate self-mastery of one's bodily functions, fluids, and abilities).

In table 2 we adapt Williams's structural dissection of film bodies for disability studies. While she focuses on the body genres of pornography, horror, and melodrama, we substitute comedy for pornography in order to apply disability to the three foundational genres of film narrative. (Of course, anomalous bodily anatomies are on display in pornography as well.) The table lists the psychic structures at play in popular Hollywood representations of disability.

From a disability studies perspective, one can readily recognize the significance of disabled bodies to the body genre formula. Rather than being based upon a generalized psychoanalytical theory, these plots depend upon the signifying affect of *disabled bodies* as a staple feature. In other words, every genre develops its own dependency on a specific disability type or two. These types then give the genres shape and coherency. They become one of the primary means by which genres become recognizable. Thus we can see the extent to which disability itself is subject to scripted social formulas for its limiting meanings. Like film plots, the disabled body itself can be said to solidify a form of visual shorthand. Its appearance prompts a finite set of interpretive possibilities now readily recognizable to audiences weaned on the grammar of visual media. Without these readable disability formulas, most body genres would be significantly hampered in their sensation-generating objectives.

Consequently, beneath comedy's common portrayal of the disabled body as out of control, the habitual monstrosity of disabled avengers, or the maimed capacity of sentimental illness drama, we find a variety of other disability subgenres, such as blind "slasher" films, which have been recycled for more than four decades now. For example, *Peeping Tom* (1960), *Wait until Dark* (1967), *Jennifer 8* (1992), *Silent Night, Deadly Night 3: Better Watch Out!* (1989), and even *Afraid of the Dark* (1991) promote identification with visually impaired, disabled female bodies in order to induce intense feel-

Table 2. An anatomy of disabled bodies in film: body genres

Genre	Comedy	Horror	Melodrama
Bodily display	faked impairment	inborn monstrosity	maimed capacity
Emotional appeal	superiority	disgust	pity
Presumed audience	men (active)	adolescent boys (active/passive)	girls/women (passive)
Disability source	performed	external	internal
Originary fantasy	sadism	sadomasochism	masochism
Resolution	humiliation	obliteration	compensation
Motivation	duplicity	revenge	restoration
Body distortion	malleability	excess	inferiority
Genre cycles	con artist, bumbling "success"	monster	long-suffering "classic"

ings (masochism) of vulnerability in an audience. The genre consistently associates femininity and visual impairment with the sensation of extreme vulnerability that the act of stalking elicits. This repeated plotline produces a web of faulty associations that threaten to turn gender and disability into synonyms for the kind of excessive vulnerability that the situation of being hunted involves. The danger here is primarily one of synecdoche whereby phenomenologies of disability and gender become synonymous with social acts of terror.

Moreover, the genre of melodrama, or the extra-tissue "weepies," focused on both male and female figures, features numerous award-winning disability vehicles, such as *The Miracle Worker* (1962), *Dark Victory* (1939), and even *Philadelphia* (1993). In these instances of disability body genres, the predominant, excessive sensation produced often hinges upon the cultivation of the fear of disability that commonly conditions audience ideas of embodiment. Such films appeal to viewer concerns about the maintenance of bodily integrity, and thus, the production of disability serves as a site of visceral sensation where abject fantasies of loss and dysfunction (maimed capacity) are made to destabilize the viewer's own investments in ability. A masochistic relationship between a suffering character and viewer vulnerability is inaugurated.

Nevertheless, these longstanding cinematic deployments of disability have remained undertheorized as a key component of all body genres. For instance, in thriller and slasher films a vengeful character with a disability is socially located as a monster. As a way of responding to socially depreciated situations, the monster secures his (sometimes her) dire need to wreak havoc on nondisabled worlds as a form of retribution for bodily loss (Longmore 1986). Such a contrivance can be witnessed as the naturalized explanation of the villain's motives in films such as *Touch of Evil* (1958), *Star Wars: Episode V—The Empire Strikes Back* (1980), *Speed* (1994), or *Richard III* (1955). In turn, audiences undergo a dual structure of identification (sado-masochism) by worrying over their own impending disablement while finding pleasure in the "hunt" as the primary sources of their identification with the imperiled victim's membership among the normative. There are myriad other combinations and permutations of these identificatory structures critical to the representation of disability, but our primary focus here is on two genres, monstrous thrillers and bumbling comedy films.

Recent examples of disabled vengeance include *Hannibal* (2001), though the title character himself is ironically exempted from this formula as a further sign of his superiority as a cultured psychotic cannibal. Hannibal's (Anthony Hopkins) psychiatric dementia is made glamorous, even titillating, in a classic disability hierarchy, by contrasting his figure to that of an even more unbearably repulsive, hyper-equipped, power-chair-using sexual deviant named Mason Verger (Gary Oldman). Audience identification is encouraged to reorient itself in favor of Hannibal-the-cannibal by getting people to root for the murderous, and more visibly obnoxious character to be dumped out of his chair and into a pit of flesh-eating hogs (and the character's personal assistant does oblige this "audience" desire). The voracious hog also figures in the family crest of the murderous disabled avenger, Richard III. Consequently, the film uses this allusion to Shakespeare—or, perhaps even more likely, to the James Bond–like retelling of the drama in Ian McKellen's film version (1995)—as a form of artistic insider lineage that helps to catapult its debased plot to the status of a psychological drama.

Similarly, examples of body genre cinema from the category of comedy, another site for disabled body viewing, also hinge upon narrow ideas about unacceptable bodies that encourage freak show–like titillation, as well as humor born of an all-too-easy superiority toward each character's bumbling incompetencies. Two such films, *Dumb and Dumberer: When Harry Met Lloyd* and *Stuck on You*, were released in 2003 with the intention of mocking special schools, "idiocy," and two guys "stuck" together, as in conjoined twins. Such cinematic products promise to heighten prior body sensation exploits by doubling and tripling the forms of abject humiliation (sadism) that the featured characters are willing to undergo, thus giving a new twist to what disability studies critic Martha Stoddard Holmes (2003) refers to as the twin structure of Victorian disability plots.

The film field, as usual, seems open to anyone—provided they can get a distributor, find corporate backing, and promise to pull in revenues. Despite

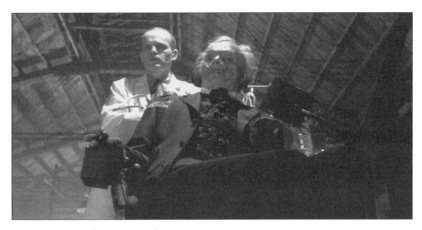

MASON VERGIL (GARY OLDMAN) AS THE DEFORMED SEXUAL DEVIANT, JUST BEFORE BEING
THROWN INTO A PIT OF HOGS BY HIS PERSONAL ASSISTANT IN
«HANNIBAL» (DIR. RIDLEY SCOTT, 2001)

this limitation, there have been some recent contemporary films that drama-
tize a canny awareness about a social model of disability. These exemplars
tend to take up disability as a core element of their storyline, as opposed to
showing a series of freak encounters. The best examples of these counter-
discursive forays include recent science fiction and comic book plots developed in *Gattaca* (1997), much of *Unbreakable* (2000), and some might
say *X-Men* (2000) and *X2: X-Men United* (2003). In these films, trite attributions of the emotional life of disabled characters—vengeance, innocence,
and barely forgivable motives born of tragedy—are swept up into a mael-
strom of disability commentary and the plight of postmodern citizenry. As
the character of Storm (Halle Berry) in *X2* points out to a new mutant:

> STORM: *They don't want us so they seek to protect us.*
> NIGHTCRAWLER: *From whom?*
> STORM: *Everyone else.*

All these films foresee a dystopic future where various incarnations of the
gene police testify to a new eugenics on the near horizon of our social context.

Mostly, though, our screens tend to transmit bizarre repetitions and standard excessive reactions to disability experience. In horror films—a genre
in which the villain is often represented as disabled—an audience's shared
sensations are not cultivated with respect to the disabled character's emotional experience. And if they are so encouraged, as in the overwrought plot
twists of Shakespeare's *Richard III* and its various theatrical and cinematic

167

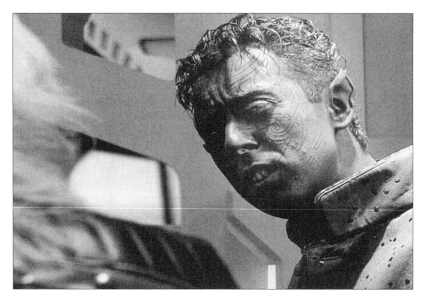

STORM (HALLE BERRY) AND NIGHTCRAWLER (ALAN CUMMING) DISCUSSING THE REASONS
FOR THE INSTITUTIONAL SEGREGATION OF MUTANTS IN «X2: X-MEN UNITED»
(DIR. BRYAN SINGER, 2003)

spinoffs, they will be eventually and gleefully exposed as an unwise audience choice. Inverse correlations to body genres occur if one goes at the topic of representation from a disability perspective: melodramas take up personal intimacy—often with a character's self-denial and repulsion toward a newly acquired disability predicament—while horror films are likely to place us in a dreadful encounter with a monstrous, but still human and disabled, character. Hence, audience experiences of sensation evoked by characters are not strictly a matter of simple identification; in the case of horror, emotions are encouraged that serve to cement longstanding associations of stigma with bodily difference.

Even so, one does not necessarily reject metaphorization while interrogating what David Wills (1995) calls "the flaw in the trope of disability." In a contest of metaphorical determinism—such as discussions of the trite "overcoming" narrative—one avoids taking refuge in an "essence" of embodied perspective. Here, disability studies is engaged in a contest of certain forms of metaphor that have dominated the historical canon of disability representations, a visceral battle over images that are not outside of questions of embodiment. Since disabled people must negotiate a finite repertoire of social meanings (both externally and internally), there are significant stakes in the humanities-based analysis of disability.

For instance, Judith Butler (1999) has argued against the existence of a prediscursive sex prior to a socially inscribed gender. She seeks not to dematerialize the embodied subjectivity of "women," but rather to privilege a discursive component to embodiment itself. Similarly, in the case of disability, we exist in our bodies by negotiating a cultural repertoire of images that threaten to mire us in debilitating narratives of dysfunction and pathology. By contesting and expanding a representational repertoire of images in culture (even by virtue of shoring up the inadequacies of our current narrative possibilities), we also create space for alternative possibilities for imagining embodied experience itself.

Just as in the key scene in *Crash* (1996), where Gabrielle (Rosanna Arquette) says, "I'd like to see if I could fit into a car designed for a normal body," disabled people are constantly negotiating a self-image with respect to a normative formula. The goal in disability studies is to leave a permanent mark upon "normative" modes of embodiment; to mar the sleek surface of normativity in the way that Gabrielle's brace buckle tears the leather bucket seat of the Mercedes without shame. A competition of image and metaphor refuses to distance audiences from the recognition that representation and embodiment are conjoined in a meaningful dependency that disability studies should not sever but deepen. In the final section of this chapter we take up recent disability documentary cinema as a site of resistance and political

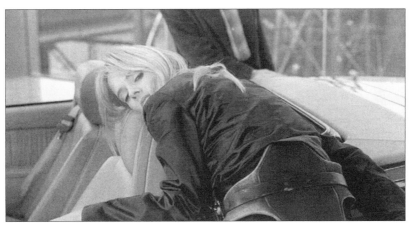

GABRIELLE (ROSANNA ARQUETTE) HUGGING A NEW CAR IN THE SHOWROOM
IN A SCENE FROM «CRASH» (DIR. DAVID CRONENBERG, 1996)

revision to the body genres discussed to this point. Our effort here is to forward these alternative film narratives as a place where competing disability subjectivities can be forged and explored.

NEW DISABILITY DOCUMENTARY CINEMA   Unlike most of the body genres, the current disability documentary cinema constitutes an avant-garde in contemporary disability depictions. Here one encounters the privileging of disabled people's voices and also the explicit foregrounding of a cultural perspective informed by, and within, the phenomenology of bodily difference. In the following discussion, we use the term *phenomenology* to mean not only the capture of disability perspectives on film, but also the meaningful influence of disability upon one's subjectivity and upon cinematic technique itself. Some recent scholars have recognized the former issue (Paterson and Hughes 1999), but we will focus on the latter, subjectivity and technique, as a means of designating the incarnation of bona fide disability cinema. Yet another site of a shift in the depiction of disability is found within subcultural communities in connection with the cultivation of disability-identified perspectives. These subcultures are in turn influenced by both international disability rights movements and the area of disability studies.

To exemplify the first point, if we step back for a moment in film history and think about U.S. film during the eugenics era, we are struck by the degree to which that era's visual film grammar assumes that an audience will be simultaneously repulsed and riveted by the display of *any* disability on screen. For instance, in the public hygiene propaganda film *Are You Fit to Marry?* (1927), near the end of the mother's dream sequence, she imagines an adult version of her disabled baby finding itself father to a strange brood of other disabled children. The pro-eugenics film takes up an explicit argument informed by beliefs about pangenesis in the nineteenth century—the belief that one kind of disability can (d)evolve into other forms of disability. While the imagined grown-up child, Claude, has something akin to cerebral palsy (a nongenetic disorder), his progeny suffer from rickets, amputations, feeblemindedness, and a host of other, unspecified malaises. One can only speculate that a psychic response cultivated in 1927 was a viewer's moral and aesthetic recoil in horror at the sight of disability begetting disability begetting disability.

But in our graduate seminar of disabled and disability studies students at the University of Illinois at Chicago, viewers tended to find the scenario ludicrous rather than repulsive. They may chuckle at the misinformed med-

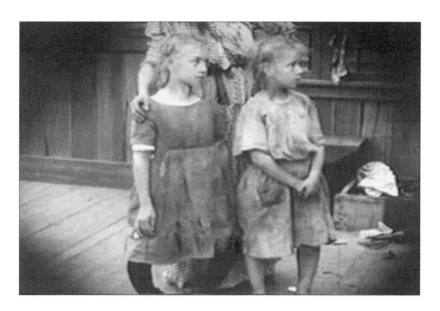

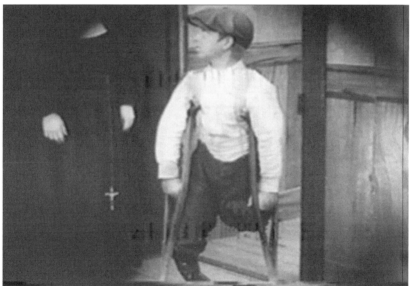

THE CONCLUDING VISION OF THE MOTHER IN «ARE YOU FIT TO MARRY?» (1927) PIVOTS ON THE
HEREDITARY TRANSMISSION OF CLAUDE LEFFINGWELL'S "DEFECTS" TO HIS CHILDREN.
BOW-LEGGEDNESS PROVIDES THE PHYSICAL VISUAL CUE TO THEIR UNSUITABILITY. (FROM
JOHN E. ALLEN ARCHIVES, NEBRASKA ETV NETWORK, QUALITY AMUSEMENT CORP.)

ical notions of an earlier decade, but mostly the students struggle to put themselves back into a mindset where the mere sight of disability is a visual rhetoric of horror and distaste. The distinction between these two audiences, one admittedly imagined and projected into the past, says a great deal about the distance one travels in a course on representations of disability and cinema. Film study challenges us not to dismiss a prior era's misinformation but, more important, to trace a long tradition of representational strategies that continue to inform cinematic technique and influence concepts of "naive" reactions to bodies. Consequently, even a film now some seventy-five years old can strike a contemporary audience as less an example of humor than a proof of the degree to which new disability cinema must take up combat with a degrading visual inheritance. Documentary, after all, just like horror, melodrama, and pornography, makes bargains to demonstrate "real life" emotions—to bring forth the most credible and empirical insider account of disability truths and existence.

In other words, a course in the history of disability cinema still brings one face to face with a sense of the wreckage left by generations of repeated representational patterns that function to the detriment of disabled people's social identity. At the same time, we study ways in which the anticipation of pleasurable information and spectacle for an audience has shifted across time.

For instance, the dream scene from *Are You Fit to Marry?* exhibits a "grotesque" fantasy about the progeny of the disabled protagonist in a series of medium shots where the mere presence of physical and cognitive disability is intended to be evidence enough of the horrible future that awaits the mother's baby if she allows him to undergo a life-saving surgery at birth. The medium shot itself suggests medical textbook photographs where an individual body is used as a stand-in for a generic disability type. Horror, in other words, is mobilized not only in the proliferation of a host of disabled bodies and the consequent social stigma that they bear, but also in the easy appeal to objectifying representational methods in medicine.

In a contemporary disability documentary, such as Diane Maroger's *Forbidden Maternity* (2002), one also gains an intimacy with many disabled characters. But in order to counter the eugenics sensation of "something gone awry" in a lineage of defective progeny, Maroger employs a variety of techniques, settings, and dramatic situations that refuse to allow audiences to take up distance, or distaste, from the presence of disabled bodies. Long shots, close-ups, and non standard framing give audiences an intimacy with disabled bodies usually reserved for private or clinical settings. In addition, Maroger shows other disabled social intimacies that the documentary's main characters, Nathalie and Bertrand, have consciously sought out as an alternative support network to a repressive familial situation.

We meet not only the two main characters, both of whom have cerebral palsy, but also their journalist friend, who also has cerebral palsy, and a host of disabled children who now occupy the institution that Nathalie and Bertrand grew up within. The film assumes a knowingness and comfort with this visual variety of bodily forms that move in and out of the alternative domestic and public space that Nathalie and Bertrand establish. The object of horror and the sadomasochistic associations that the genre traditionally employs are directly inverted in new disability documentary cinema since the audience is situated to respond with revulsion at the debasing mindset that dominates the characters' interactions with an able-bodied world. While the proselytizers of the eugenics period denoted the disabled body as the objectionable object within a sea of normalcy, new disability documentary cinema designates degrading social contexts as that which need to be rehabilitated.

But a mindset is often difficult to depict, particularly when one seeks to designate a generalized and amorphous dominant perspective about people with disabilities—one that is ubiquitous and yet evident only through documents, investigations, and paperwork, which must be compiled and pieced together over the course of a lifetime. Surely, as Mark Sherry has demonstrated, disability hate crime does exist (2000), but many of the serious troubles of disability existence can only be put together through the series of deflections, distrust, and disavowals reserved for disabled bodies in apparently separate and contingent moments of excessive interventions and discrimination.

By and large, in its depiction of Bertrand and Nathalie's life, *Forbidden Maternity* lingers on details that might seem inconsequential. For example, near the middle of the film there is an extended scene shot in the kitchen of their apartment where Bertrand makes salad with a friend who has come over to share dinner with the couple. While Hollywood would rarely "waste" footage in the recording of such a seemingly innocuous scenario, *Forbidden Maternity* recognizes that one of its main oppositions is the mainstream belief that disabled people are unduly dependent and cannot manage the details of ordinary domestic life. For example, salad mixing, without some gut-wrenching and dramatic circumstance going on around it, would end up on the cutting-room floor of most Hollywood productions. In disability documentary cinema this kind of detail must be captured as the essence of the argument.

In many ways these films function as the empirical evidence, captured visually, that sets out to refute scientific formulas about the management of disability and the false reliance on a myth of personal independence. The day-to-day details *are the point* because it is at this most basic level of modern existence that bureaucracies have doubted the ability of people with disabilities to manage their own affairs. In this sense, the new documentary disability cinema's focus on singular case studies opposes much of today's science on disability, which seeks to generalize management and control schemes for disabled multitudes—who are all discounted from the start from being able to coexist with their nondisabled peers. Such a context of systemic doubt and suspicion entails scenes that ask people with mobility impairments to perform their walking gait as "proof" that they need a handicap parking ticket.

Such a point can also be found in a video such as *When Billy Broke His Head* (1995), in which the filmmaker-narrator (Billy Golfus), who has recently experienced a traumatic brain injury, visits disabled activists and community members who suddenly populate his social landscape with a variety of previously unfamiliar disability perspectives. For instance, we visit the disabled musician Larry Kegan, who shares the details of his personal dressing habits with the protagonist, and by extension his audience, as a way of underscoring the complex negotiation of even the most routine rituals of everyday life. Or we drive with Billy next to a woman with a neurological disability who navigates the streets of her hometown in her specially equipped van with "only one minor traffic ticket in nine years." Such incidents significantly parallel the salad mixing scene in *Forbidden Maternity*, in that they portray disabled people engaged in common activities that become extraordinarily uncommon, and even unlikely, within societies that seek to restrain, segregate, and institutionalize disabled people on the basis of their differences.

When viewers enter into these new disability documentary media landscapes, they discover immediately that routine activities refute the opposition to disabled people's freedom as a denial of the right to pursue lives that are recognizably ordinary. For a generation weaned on spectacular images, gravity-defying special effects, and the digitized erasure of appendages, the new landscape of disability documentary at first may seem anything but "spectacular" in comparison to the well-worn formulas of body genres. These films unfold arguments that demand a focus upon activities that have been all but ousted from traditional Hollywood fare. The new disability documentary cinema strives, first and foremost, to make an ordinary life with disability imaginable and even palatable to a society that holds a bankrupt tradition of disability imagery. This demand upon the audiences of new disability documentary cinema involves what the cultural critic Michael Ventura explains as the imaginative leap of identifying with a character who is not "conventionally beautiful": "But the face of Helen Keller was marked by her enormous powers of concentration, while to cast the face of Mare Winningham [who played Helen Keller] in the role is to suggest, powerfully, that one can come back from the depths unscathed. No small delusion is being sold here" (1988, 177).

Singular portrayals of people with disabilities are a staple and contrivance of popular genre filmmaking. In genre films, an audience consumes representations of disability one character at a time and most often follows that lone figure into an either/or resolution of death or cure ("the only two acceptable states," according to the disabled writer Anne Finger [1997, 257]). In contrast, new disability documentary cinema seeks to counter with the portrayal of disability ensembles.

One could argue that the primary convention of this new documentary genre is the effort to turn disability into a chorus of perspectives that deepen and multiply narrow cultural labels that often imprison disabled people within taxonomic medical categories. The medical model specifies a generalized body type that can presumably be true for all bodies within a classificatory rubric of disorder. While disability documentary films do not seek to repress, suppress, or erase the fact of differing biological capacities and appearances (as is sometimes charged in critiques of disability studies), they do seek to refute pathological classifications that prove too narrow and limiting to encompass an entire human life as it is *lived*. For instance, in *Forbidden Maternity* Bertrand and Nathalie's disabled journalist friend explains:

> As a person with C.P. I've always had to fight to explain those two letters that were my two letters—the letters that qualified me and always required an explanation. People could see I was disabled. I was obviously mobility impaired given the way my legs were. But when I mentioned "cerebral," they'd say, "cerebral? From the way you speak one wouldn't guess you're *cerebrally* handicapped." So I'd say, "I'm not cerebrally handicapped. I have cerebral palsy. In other words, when I was born my brain was wounded and this had consequences. In my case, this resulted in walking difficulties. In another person with C.P. it may result in speech impediment or trouble using the hands. That's what *cerebral* means. I never said *mental*. It seems to me you're confusing the words *cerebral* and *mental*."

To confuse the word *cerebral* with *mental* is to attempt to malign one form of disability with another. Conditions become stigmatized when we allow attributes to endlessly bleed into further disorders. Thus, disability exists on a lethal medicalized continuum where ascriptions of inferiority deepen and further disqualify bodies.

As a result, people with physical disabilities find themselves refuting cognitive "involvements" (as in the case of cerebral palsy), and, in turn, people with cognitive disabilities find themselves having to charge those with physical disabilities with a further sedimenting of their own socially derived stigma. In either case the effort is futile because the fates of both groups are historically tethered to each other. Eugenics beliefs used physical disabilities and deformities to reference the "feeblemindedness" residing within, and those who tested below a certain IQ level found themselves standing naked in front of medical personnel searching for the inevitable physical stigmata (Snyder and Mitchell 2002). Today, those most likely to be institutionalized, as Frederick Wiseman's Multi-handicapped Series shows, are consistently designated as residing among the "multiply disabled."

While it may seem surprising or even odd to be rehearsing the diagnostic fine points of the multiple permutations of individual experience of a disorder (in a particular environment enfolding a particular body), the new disability documentary cinema does not refuse impairment (as many contend even in disability studies) (Finkelstein 1996; Shakespeare 1997; Barnes 1999). Rather, these films insist on recognition of a more complex human constellation of experiences that inform medical categories such as cerebral palsy. One must essentially explode the classification's rigid yet often amorphous parameters in order to recognize a more multiple and variegated existence within its boundaries.

In our own documentary video *Vital Signs: Crip Culture Talks Back* (1995), a similar principle is at stake. Rather than foreground a singular voice capable of refuting the inhumanity and derision that disabled people associate with their most inconsequential social interactions, the video orchestrates multiple disability perspectives to represent what used to be inaccurately referred to as "the disability experience." The point of the film is not merely to present a chorus of voices but to capture the diversity, originality, and vitality of vantage points that characterize contemporary disability communities. Thus, when the disabled performance artist Cheryl Marie Wade says that "they can have their little telethons as long as we are on there [the television] doing all the other things we do," an alternative perspective from Bob DeFelice promptly counters that "I love telethons. I absolutely love them!" Like all vibrant subcultures, disability culture is diffuse and orchestrates multiple perspectives, as well as bodies, somatic systems, and minds.

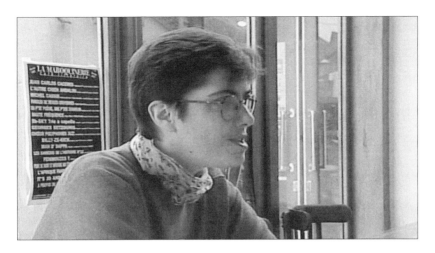

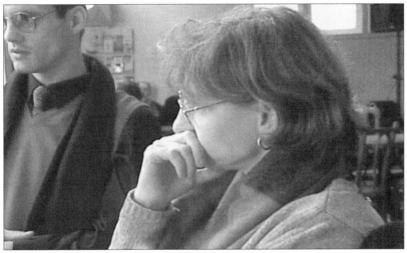

CP DISCUSSION IN LUNCHROOM WITH BERTRAND, NATHALIE, AND THEIR JOURNALIST FRIEND, FROM «FORBIDDEN MATERNITY» (DIR. DIANE MAROGER, 2002)

After a showing of *Vital Signs* at a conference of special educators in Chicago, the first respondent in the audience exclaimed, "Wow! All of those people are so articulate and in control of their life stories. They're nothing like the disabled people that we see in classes everyday." After mulling over the meaning of the comment, we realized the point was that the video paraded a somewhat idiosyncratic and articulate group of disabled people who diverge wildly from the students who populate special education classes across the country. In response, we argued that disability documentary cinema was not

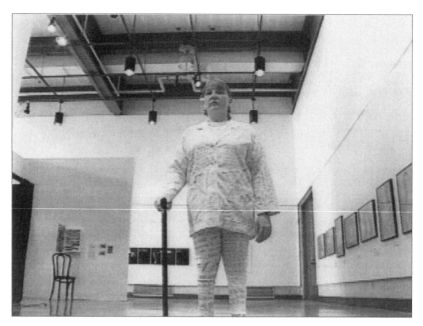

CARRIE SANDAHL'S PERFORMANCE IN «VITAL SIGNS: CRIP CULTURE TALKS BACK»
(DIR. SHARON SNYDER, 1995)

about showcasing a transcendent point of view but rather is a visceral rewriting of the way that we understand disability. The subject of *Vital Signs* is not the singular insights of atypical disabled people, but rather the creativity that sparks and energizes disabled people when they find themselves in a community of their peers, performing their knowledge and strategies for an audience that is anxious to learn the fine points of social negotiation in such hostile environments.

What shifts most radically in this scenario is not the persons depicted, but the way one comprehends disability experience as fuel for creativity—as opposed to tragedy, burden, or misfortune. The new disability documentary cinema changes the terms upon which our understanding of disability experience rests. In *Vital Signs* the Irish disabled performance artist, Mary Duffy, explains this dilemma: "Most people approach me as if [to say] you're a walking, talking disabled person. You're not supposed to talk back." The social expectations of disabled people are often so low that even the most cursory interaction promotes shock and disbelief. But the documentary is charged with instilling a new narrative pleasure: disabled persons such as Mary Duffy, offering disability-based insights and her own body/life's exemplarity of it.

Another comment at the special education conference came from teachers who worried about showing the film to their students for fear that disabled youngsters would be turned off by being pegged as the "expert" on disability experience. As if they hadn't already been defined as detrimentally different within the normative classroom of most educational settings! In other words, the expressed concern was largely one that struggles with what it means to be singled out and stigmatized for a difference that has been noticed but not openly discussed. What if individual students have acquired a range of knowledge and experience that the teacher lacks? Our own approach to this issue is that without adequate pedagogical contexts about disability history and experience, such as those available in the new disability documentary cinema, disabled students will continue to drift and to perform below many of their nondisabled peers. In recent surveys of disabled students' achievement in U.S. public education, only students with a developed disabled identity manage to perform at or above the academic level of nondisabled students. Such a fact calls out for a change in our public school curriculums that continue to erase disability content from the canon of Western culture. Just as female students and students of color tend to flourish in educational settings that promote the insights of their own communities in history, disabled students will continue to find education largely irrelevant as long as it sidelines their experiences and body differences as insignificant or irrelevant.

CINEMATIC INTERVENTIONS   In closing, we return briefly to our discussion of disability in historical context. One of the primary insights gained from study of the eugenics era was that disability proved to be a uniquely modern phenomenon: we had orchestrated a culture so fast moving, complex, and demanding that many bodies could not adequately keep up. Yet, despite this accurate depiction of contemporary modern life, the fatal flaw in eugenics theory was that, rather than targeting the social context as something in need of repair, it singled out the disabled bodies themselves as the targeted sites of intervention. Thus, efforts at cure, rehabilitation, segregation, prevention—even extermination—dominate the various eugenics approaches toward disabled bodies. Disabled bodies were at the forefront of modern innovation, in their experience of intervention upon the body as a primary means of redress.

Popular film genres developed by sporting a host of interventions to alleviate individual bodies of their socially derived stigma. In 1950 Marlon Brando had his first starring role in *The Men*, which featured the wonders of a new rehabilitation industry that could successfully adjust even the paraplegic's incapacitated body; in the 1970s a spate of returning-veterans films foregrounded sex as the root of an appropriate personal adjustment to post-war disability. Melodramas such as *Forrest Gump* (1994) miraculously repair the bodies of double amputees as a solution to the conundrum that disability has been made to present. And horror films such as *Hannibal* promote the expendability of physically disabled bodies relative to the more fashionable and cultured exploits of "psychotic" cannibalism. All these films trade upon a dominant opposition in the post-eugenics period that is involved in extreme efforts to fix disabled people in order to relieve society of the need to be more inclusive and accommodating of difference.

In contrast, the new disability documentary cinema seeks to target the rightful site of meaningful intervention: namely, a lethal and brutal social context. Rather than identifying different bodies as the appropriate locus of intervention, these works target uncomprehending social systems as a necessary domain of social commentary in film. They foreground disabled bodies while interrogating contemporary social management systems that seek to survey, manage, and control nearly every aspect of their existence. New disability documentary cinema captures uncomprehending interactions between disabled persons and the bureaucracies that ensnare them. In *Forbidden Maternity*, Bertrand and Nathalie must solicit the help of a social worker in order to refute their institutional records that portray both of them as victims of "profound mental deficiencies." In *When Billy Broke His Head*, the narrator must show up at the welfare office in person to get his reduced Social Security checks reinstated to the paltry amount of $522 per month. In *Vital Signs* disabled artists turn their objectifying experiences within the medical industry into social commentaries about the eradication of their humanity in medical theaters and clinical settings.

These films tend to target those institutions that were initially designed to accommodate disability's "endless" differences. Instead of flexible systems, contemporary institutions reveal themselves as monolithic entities that direct all the details of people's existence. They become equal-opportunity sites of discrimination that extract disabled people from pursuing their lives by burying them in a morass of legalistic and bureaucratic paperwork. When viewed collectively, these films give the sense that our post-eugenic era specializes in keeping disabled people busy so that they demand less of the outside world as active participants.

This is a wholly different take than the other world of body genres where people don't want to have their pleasures politicized. All the films that return disabled charges to institutions—or worse, offer euthanasia—as a meaningful resolution (including films with spectacular and complex disability-identified perspectives, such as *One Flew over the Cuckoo's Nest* [1975], *Rain Man* [1988], *Girl, Interrupted* [1999]) summon up assurances about the beneficence of therapists, modern social organizations, and incarcerating stone walls beneath "soothing" adobe façades. Most disability narratives, however experimental, end up trying to prove that every white coat means well in returning us to safekeeping—on screen, through a window, where we witness disability experiences managed by comfortable quarters, as if filmed through a soft focus filter. Such a patronizing impulse is well characterized at the conclusion of *Minority Report* (2002) when the protagonist (Tom Cruise) whisks off his autistic female charge for safekeeping on an island. There, presumably, she will both be shielded from the incomprehensions and exploitative tendencies of able-bodied culture, while also finding her feminine passivity redeemed by his sexual interest. It is in film that we encounter disability largely as a "plight to be conquered"—as long as, when the lights come up, we don't find the same bodies blocking the aisles on our way back to the theater lobby.

Part III

INSTITUTIONALIZING DISABILITY STUDIES

SIX

Conclusion | *Compulsory*
Feral-ization

This final chapter examines the status of the field of disability studies as it becomes formally institutionalized in the contemporary American university. While disability studies has opened up new discursive spaces for revising cultural attitudes and beliefs about disability, its increasing legitimation within the academy comes with its own conflicts. The university as a research location cannot merely divorce itself from the ethical and restrictive practices that have characterized the treatment of disabled people during the past two centuries. The institutionalization of disability studies is just that—a formal cultural ingestion process that churns out more knowledge about disability while resisting reflexive inquiries about whether or not more is inherently better. Of course, more knowledge is better for the institution because it keeps the research mill active, but here we want to contemplate the degree to which an increase in disability-based data threatens to reproduce some of the problems discussed in the chapters of this book.

The title of this chapter belongs to one of our Ph.D. students, Bruce Henderson, who introduced it during a graduate seminar on disability, eugenics, and evolution. By "compulsory feral-ization," he may have intended both to play upon the early twentieth-century practice of compulsory sterilization and to suggest how disabilities tend to be automatically turned into examples of human insufficiencies in need of professional mediation. Within this scenario disability becomes a throwback to a prior, subhuman state. Disabled people often contest this association of their bodies with lack. For instance, in a recent correspondence the "Cuckoo" comic book artist Madison Clell argued, "I *strongly* disagree that Dissociative Identity Disorder [multiple personality disorder] is a disability—it can become disabling for day to day functioning but in reality its genesis is an efficient survival mechanism" (personal communication, 6 February 2004). Beyond this refusal to see disability as synonymous with pathology, the phrase "compulsory feral-ization" also suggests that the history of disability has continued to resonate with early efforts in France to *train* the wild boy of Aveyron—he who was christened with the label "feral child" and stood for a whole line of savage children reared in nature by wolves and other nonhuman creatures.[1]

The feral child was an invention of post-Enlightenment Europe—a kind of collective mirage that, as in the early days of colonialism, presented an opportunity to conquer a lost primitive human self. The category—for it served more as an orchestrating classification of medical science than as a description of individual behavior—brought together myth and empiricism by associating a child who was deaf, mute, and perhaps autistic, with a condition that represented both a form of subhumanity and a radical humanitarian promise. The feral child was recognized as a disadvantaged entity cut off from the civilizing efforts of human communities, what the renowned mental asylum reformer Pinel called an "incurable idiot" (Shattuck 1980, 37). Efforts to educate feral children set into motion the elaborate apparatus around "idiocy" that culminated in the field of eugenics. Yet this dismissive and dehumanizing diagnosis of the "wild boy" was tempered by psychologists such as Itard and Séguin who saw him as a potential link to an unadulterated human nature to which moderns had lost access. This savage existence represented the opportunity to test out the Romantic notion of individuals as blank slates—a surface upon which culture inscribed itself in shaping a self. The wild boy, later named Victor by Itard because of his presumed liking for the sound of the vowel *o*, promised to solidify pre-Darwinian theories of evolution. This combination of failed humanity and primitive hope may seem paradoxical. But if we recognize these two descriptions as a general formula for disability, then "compulsory feral-ization" nicely sums up the situation: historically disability has represented both an example of faulty human organisms and the promise of a body that might teach us something about "ourselves" (noting that "ourselves" does not include people with disabilities).[2]

In either scenario, the critical terrain shared is one of research and its inevitable byproduct, intervention. As an example of organic failure or insufficiency, disability, by definition, embodies the need for compensation; the sciences situate disability either as a functional deficit in need of restoration or as a failure of the social context to adequately accommodate difference. As an example of "primitive promise," disability is situated as an opportunity to learn about ourselves as vulnerable organisms—the reestablishment of our own bodies to some "rudimentary origin" where the mechanics of the organism were somehow more self-evident. Thus disability is recognized essentially as a *body-in-the-making*. As the bald, albino, female protagonist/narrator, Olympia, in Dunn's *Geek Love* explains, "There's something about disability that's like wearing your vulnerability on your sleeve, as if all of my secrets are exposed, and people trust in me enough to confess their own secrets of failure or dysfunction." Disabled bodies represent a potential valuable source of information about generic organicity, while also finding themselves shut out of meaningful communion with others. As long as disability is narrated in this way, disabled people will be the objects of an inexhaustible research machine—one that wantonly uses up their bodies, their energies, and their time. One of the primary oppressions experienced by disabled people is that they are marked as perpetually available for all kinds of intrusions, both public and private. Disability makes one's body fodder for any number of invasive approaches.

This was true for feral children as well.[3] Their savagery or wildness justified incarceration, disciplinary regulation, experimentation, and, ultimately, abandonment by the professions presumably devoted to their salvage. For Itard, Victor represented both an opportunity and an impossibility. Here is how Michael Newton (2003) characterizes their relationship after years of intervention could not bring Victor to speak:

> It is not hard to feel as sorry for Itard as one feels for the wild child. For Victor's story catches hold of a vivid and tactful tenderness: its subject is ultimately that of yearning for and missing love. Unwittingly, perhaps, Itard left us a story not just of the education of a young savage, but of his own inability to be close or intimate. A scientific detachment operates in Itard, and he watches with surprise and regret as the emotions he obviously feels for Victor are hardly reciprocated. . . . Itard seems doomed to detach himself from those he tried to get close to. Pupil and teacher, father and son, adult and child, doctor and patient,

scientist and subject—in each case the relationship is skewed and fundamentally unequal. Itard clearly dreamed of rescue for the young and abandoned boy. Some lost part of himself must have seemed contained in poor Victor, something that he might retrieve, look after and make better. Yet the imbalance of power between the two of them, the unbridgeable distance between their several worlds, doomed the attempt; and in the end, it is Victor, the named one, who haunts us as he haunted Itard. (127)

We think this description by Newton gets the conflict exactly right in many ways. Ultimately, the record of Victor functions as little more than a Western empiricist's fantasy. The story of the wild boy is the story of Itard's own personal and professional failure to bridge a gap that Victor refuses. He becomes the quintessential unwilling subject with respect to the goals of scientific research, in that he will not be interpolated into the discourse of "rescue." Whose desire is on display here? Is it Victor's need to have intercourse with a civil society that would exhibit and pander to his "savagery," or that of Itard, the surrogate of science, who "dreams" of access to the "wild boy's savage secrets" on behalf of his own professional reputation.

Within this scenario, disability finds itself in a peculiar situation in the institution of the academy, where it is allied with a form of subaltern knowledge that is both disparaged and sought after at the same time. Research invests itself with the promise of solving the riddle of human differences while undermining the humanity of its object of study with a chivalric story of rescue. Ultimately, as Gayatri Spivak (1988, 287) and Homi Bhabha (1994, 116) both point out, the exotic object of academic study must be constituted not as an undifferentiated monolith, but rather as a *hybridized* (or, in Spivak's terms, irreducibly differentiated) identity.[4] This is so particularly if the term *hybridization* is understood to mean "less than one and double" (Bhabha 1994, 116), an object ceaselessly divided across multiple categories yet somehow less human at the same time. This formulation of the subaltern is critical to a new understanding of disability. We are not talking about power's violent suppression of its object, but rather the situation of disability as something to be "solved" and then perpetually returned to its cultural location of mystery. Disability is that which is endlessly differentiated into myriad categories of dysfunction yet never made coherent (or, you might say, successfully "cured" of its defining difference).

This subaltern status, we would argue, significantly describes the situation not only of disabled people but also of disability studies in the academy today. The historical treatment of disabled people has come home to roost in the contemporary location of disability studies in the university. Just as

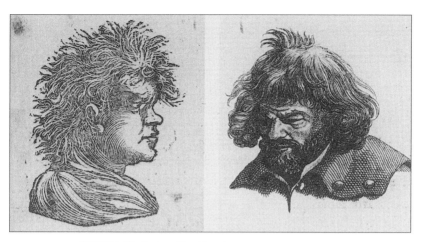

THE WILD BOY OF AVEYRON, AS A YOUTH AND AS AN OLDER MAN

Itard longed for a more meaningful relationship with Victor, disability studies seems to provoke a similar response from those disciplines most dependent upon narratives of disability as insufficiency in need of normalization (special education, physical therapy, occupational therapy, communication disorders, nursing, medicine, kinesiology). In other words, compulsory feralization. Disability studies is recognized as both a threat and a saving grace of sorts among the health sciences. It represents a threat in the sense of a once silenced object now given the agency to talk back to the professions that would speak its inferiority; a saving grace in that the inclusion of disabled people in any meaningful way suggests fields that are beyond reproach in their humanitarian commitments. The rehabilitation sciences yearn to be accepted in the field of disability studies. But that longing is tempered by some significant hostility toward disabled people and disability-identified scholars, who are now perceived as controlling the terms of the rehabilitation sciences' participation in disability studies. This compensatory desire is literal in the sense of an earnest belief in "helping" disabled people as a primary value, and visceral as a commitment to mending (or, at least, disguising) bodies believed to violate socially or scientifically devised norms of appearance and functionality.

There is a foundational impulse across the sciences and therapies to treat disability as something gone awry—to tame the "wildness" that bodily, sensory, and cognitive differences represent. As one faculty member in physical therapy at a large midwestern university argued, "We are here to *help* disabled people with their problems." Yet helping does not extend to seeking disabled people's input as to what they want from therapy, nor does it envision the possibility that disabled people might want to be trained as physical therapists themselves. There has been a longstanding assumption by some in the field of physical therapy that disabled people cannot perform the physical (and, perhaps, intellectual?) demands of the profession. Yet physical therapy programs in other countries, such as the program at the University of Costa Rica, are training individuals with disabilities as future practitioners. The investment in practices of assistance toward disabled people is honestly "deep," but also riddled with ambivalence—that which Newton refers to as a doomed detachment toward those one seeks to save. Its objectifying premise is the need to cure, disguise, or lessen the difference that marks the clientele as faulty. Therefore, the thing that made the "feral child" desirable—its primitive deviance, if you will—can be accessed only by its own destruction. Similarly, disability draws the attentions of fields that seek to cure, fix, repair, or deny its existence. *Disability is a difference that exists only to be undone.*

Let us explain how we understand the field, in order to draw the parallels necessary to make this paradoxical formula of compulsory feral-ization meaningful. Particularly as we try to imagine the role of disability studies among the ranks of other legitimated academic disciplines. As a celebrated case study, disability studies, ironically, fills its role as an exceptional, albeit unruly, child. Of course, no one wants to qualify as an "exceptional child" if that means a "special" exception in need of various qualifiers, a lowering of standards, and infantilizing treatment. Harlan Hahn refers to this tendency in our video *Vital Signs: Crip Culture Talks Back* (1995) as a distaste for euphemism: as if "disability were so awful that you have to disguise it with all of these fancy words. We [the disability community] don't like that!" During his time in Paris, the wild boy Victor was singled out for a great deal of "special treatment," such as having a battery affixed to his person that administered electric shocks for bad behavior; undergoing numerous psychological and physiological tests for the assessment of his functional status as a throwback; and being hung out of a fourth story window by his feet in order to better align his interests with the goals of his "training." These curious signs of commitment to Victor's well-being reflect the desperation that his managers felt at forging a direct relationship between their imagined object of study and the one that was actually before them.

What became immediately obvious—and this is the danger of having one's object of research suddenly *on location*—is that there existed considerable distance between Victor's desires (whatever those might have been) and those of the diagnostic institution. The Jamaican writer Michelle Cliff explains her identification with the "wild boy" as a Jamaican subject of British colonialism in her essay "A Journey into Speech" (1988): "I felt, with Victor, that my wildness had been tamed—that which I had been taught was my wildness" (57). In other words, not only was Victor being trained in the manners and customs of the moderns, he was also being taught his savagery—a barbarism that he himself had not recognized before he was ingested in the classification of "feral."

This same situation of oppositions has, to some degree, characterized efforts to integrate disability studies into the contemporary university. As various programs in disability studies find their way into academia, the field itself functions as a form of disciplinary case study for other institutions and the disability community in general. While no one in the field has been subjected to electrical shock or hung out of a fourth floor window by his or her feet (at least so far as we know), disability studies faculty and students endlessly feel the press of the object ensconced within the very institution to which it has dedicated its critique. Thus, like Victor, we are being taught our wildness to the degree that the perspective of disability studies proves so difficult to institutionalize. For instance, almost as a literalization of its disciplinary location, the disability studies program in one large midwestern university exists precariously beside the therapies and medical school on one side and public health on the other. This physical locale places many disabled people on campus in proximity to practitioners in these other fields. Disabled students, staff, and faculty pass white-coated individuals on the sidewalk fairly regularly, and often the white-coated strollers crane their necks for a quick diagnostic assessment of the bodies making their way through an inaccessible, urban campus. One can be diagnosed many times when sharing pathways (both textual and literal) with medical and rehabilitation professionals. Just as Victor was unleashed into the courtyard at the Institute for Deaf-Mutes for Parisians to gawk at him, so one can find oneself the subject of evaluating gazes with some frequency at universities that train medical and rehabilitation professionals.

As a result of this physical arrangement of campus buildings and the fact that therapy students make up a portion of the disability studies graduate student cohort, some therapy students have reported feeling "unnerved" by the privileging of disability perspectives within disability studies—even when students in the program advocate nothing more radical than the need to make the therapies more responsive to disabled people's goals. These professions have always imagined their commitment to disabled people as their primary value, and hearing that disabled people—particularly those in disability studies—do not necessarily share this sentiment often comes as a shock. The revelation rocks the foundation of these applied disciplines and necessitates a reorientation on the part of the practitioners. Some faculty in the therapeutic sciences have commented that as their students come into contact with disability studies courses, faculty, and students, they often feel alienated and contemplate dropping out of such programs. The claim references a lack of academic comfort as therapy students embark on their studies, and the result is a feeling that they do not belong conceptually to disability studies. In these comments disability studies is often represented as hostile ideological territory for some of those trained in the therapeutic sciences.

As a result, disability studies finds itself saddled with an expectation to make therapy students feel "comfortable," even though the discipline often traffics in the discomforting challenge of many personal and public perspectives about human differences; in order to belong conceptually to disability studies, the therapies have consistently argued that the rehabilitation of deficient bodies must be included in the field. In addition, researchers in the therapies argue that impairment-based research should be included in a broad conceptualization of disability studies. Conceding these approaches to disability as part of disability studies would be tantamount to acknowledging one's own internalization of deviance—to speak one's own subjugation on a bodily continuum from superior to normal to aberrant. This effort to have disabled clients speak their own debasement (even if this means positing their own state of mind for them) has been the ultimate goal of disciplines seeking to justify their own efforts. Here we come directly into contact with the advent of compulsory feral-ization: as with disability culture, disability studies must be tamed because it is undisciplined and, as one *New York Times* article (Martin 1997) put it, would "bite the hands that would feed [it]." Newton tells how Victor grows so frustrated by his efforts to have his desires recognized as legitimate that he viciously bites Itard's hand (2003, 125).

The institutionalization of disability studies comes fraught with difficulties in that the field situates itself as a force of destabilization—one that would undermine historical efforts on behalf of individual insufficiencies by displacing the object of change onto unaccommodating environments, beliefs, disciplines, or research methods.

TAXING BODIES OF RESEARCH One of the most pressing questions for administrators, faculty, and disability communities participating in the establishment of courses or degree programs in disability studies concerns research. While the power inequities that mark race, gender, and sexuality have been often characterized with respect to a lack of attention to the particularities of marginalized bodies and their unique cultural circumstances, the oppression of disabled people has occurred as a result of their perpetual identification as an object of research. This distinction points to the ways in which disability differs from other minority locations, while also suggesting that its intersection with race, gender, and sexuality may fill in critical gaps in the current knowledge base of disability studies.

Disability history has been marked by the overindulgence of the medical sciences and therapies in the scrutiny of "biological" differences. From the sixteenth-century practice of collecting catalogues of monsters and marvels to today's search for genetic codes of deviance, disabled people have served as the relics of obscene curiosity disguised beneath the neutral veil of empirical inquiry. As a result, disabled people have been objectified within classifications of deviance, but this objectification, we would argue, is neither the sole nor perhaps even the primary source of disability oppression at the hands of the diagnostic sciences. Instead, we must turn our attention to what we might call "the exhaustion of people-based research practices," where disabled individuals' time, liberty, and energies are expended without concern or adequate caution. The trajectory of history with respect to disabled people shows an increasing tendency to restrict freedoms through the disregard of time as a commodity of value in lives marked as "disabled."

Foucault spent much of his research career arguing that excessive diagnosis and the evaluation of bodies within categories of pathology proved to be the characteristic form of oppression in the modern period. This period also saw the rise and professionalization of medicine and later the rehabilitation sciences. The science of bodies evolved (or devolved, depending on your point of view) from a descriptive effort to empirically record instances of human variation toward an increasingly judgmental classification of bodies among hierarchies of deviance. Medical science thereby effectively surrendered its claims to practice objective methodologies. Rather than charting bodies as diverse entities interacting with and adapting to their external and internal environments, medicine developed an increasingly abstract notion of the "ideal" body founded upon the statistical evaluation of norms. In addition, science sought to measure and monitor bodies as discrete materials divorced from their social, historical, and environmental contexts. As we have argued, the feral child was continually located within the annals of myth where children were raised by animals rather than being seen as the product of, say, parental disregard, communal ostracism, or violent scapegoating.[5]

People with disabilities recognize the oppressive force of diagnosis and evaluation all too viscerally, for many have spent their lives beneath the judgmental surveillance of medical and rehabilitation regimes. For instance, during lectures to medical students we often ask how many know the empirical classifications for cognitive disabilities at the turn of the twentieth century. No medical students ever seems to know the answer to this question because, as the intellectual historian John Limon argues, medicine (like other sciences) tends to cannibalize its own past in the name of progress (1990, 9). When we explain that the accurate answer is "idiot, imbecile, moron, and subnormal (with moron and subnormal existing at the more 'advanced' end of the spectrum)," medical students act either amazed or embarrassedly amused. Even without knowing the historical etymology of these words as diagnoses, they are all quite familiar with the terms. Clearly, medical terminology of this sort is not value-neutral and often reflects the prejudices of those who purvey such classifications as empirical knowledge.

If Victor was referred to as "a profound idiot," or as "subhuman," or as "afflicted with the intransigence of the deaf and mute," these terms are misrecognized if we do not understand the misanthropy that informs them. They are not value-free classifications used in a merely descriptive fashion in their time. Rather, they embody attitudes of the historical moment in which they were produced. The informing attitudes behind such designations give way to the torpor that makes them available later as childhood taunts. In using once scientific classifications such as these, we access and expose the venom underlying their originary formation in pathologizing rhetoric. In some ways, one could as easily argue that these terms become effective slanders in the public realm because they falsely posed as empirical when they were used as professional diagnoses in an earlier moment. We do not appropriate these terms as derogatory as an exercise in ahistoricism or decontextualization. Their availability as pejorative rhetoric was always already embodied in their initial usage within medicine and rehabilitation.

INSTITUTIONALIZING DISABILITY STUDIES In keeping with this critique of knowledge formation and linguistic determinism, Foucault ultimately extended his criticism to the academy for participating in the post-Enlightenment press of developing research data that would deliver a tangible, even politicized, knowledge of bodies and their attendant pathologies to the "light" of academic disciplines. All of this has a bearing for disability research practices today devoted to the administration of disability in higher education and the attendant development of "new" research strategies in the academy as a contemporary location of disability. Is it possible to keep the freshness—the insight-driven "wildness"—of the field in the midst of seeking a home base in the academy? Can disability studies sustain its productive "feral" nature without being reduced to a lesser form of academic evolutionism or thoroughly domesticated as an academic endeavor?

To navigate this difficult line between professionalization and revolutionary invention, those of us in disability studies must ask the following question of ourselves: How can we cultivate and continue to pursue research about disability without further subjugating an overanalyzed and diagnosed population? Can disability studies and the study of disability pursue work without further contributing to the oppression of those bodies that researchers seek to know and assess—even liberate? What lessons must we take from a history of "people-based research practices" performed in the name of disabled peoples' best interests? Can we avert the practice of compulsory feral-ization even as we espouse radical schemes of critique?

Profoundly important questions await the cultivation of the field within the academy—questions that disability venues and university faculty developing disability-based courses and programs need to take up in a forthright and meaningful way. The successful retention of the field's "freshness" depends a great deal on maintaining proximity to the struggles of local disability communities—both political and arts-based. If one pursues one's existence outside of the formalities of the academy, political and perspectival orthodoxies are less likely to pass as disinterested. Consequently, maintenance of proximity to non–academically based disability communities provides a critical formula for keeping an "edge" to the disability studies research agenda. Like Victor, disability studies can have its "wildness" taught to it and trained out of it. While some of the forces of institutional "domestication" are bound to set in, the field needs to consciously cultivate its roots in activist communities to retain a degree of necessary "wildness."

In some disability studies programs, local disability communities continue to play a pivotal role in policing the university. They are especially vigilant in reminding researchers of their penchant for overassessment and the rampant disregard of disabled people's time and energy—that which we have designated as the "exhaustion of people-based research practices." Moreover, disabled people's information gives researchers privileged access to vital and unique perspectives; thus, subjects with disabilities should receive meaningful compensation, as do other groups of research subjects. Private industry has recognized this form of exploitation to a much greater degree than the university. The practice of well-paid researchers paying their subjects only a token amount for their participation must come to an end. Here we will give some examples from the contemporary institutionalization of disability in the academy as an area of critical inquiry. These examples represent a way to envision the project of disability studies more fully, if we can champion the continuing study of disability in an ethical manner.

In part, disability studies must recognize that its critique should be trained on the institution of the academy as much as on the social and political context outside its walls. By being situated within universities that also host the health sciences, for instance, disability studies inevitably comes into contact with those disciplines focusing on impairment-based research; it thus "violates" a longstanding injunction within social model approaches to disability with regard to ignoring questions of impairment. Impairment—that is, characteristics linked to an underlying physiological deficit that prevent a person from performing (or appearing) typically—is very much part of the analytical terrain that U.S. models of disability studies take up. By and large, the study of impairment continues in medicine and the therapies as an objectifying practice with respect to the designation of disability as pathology; however, in U.S. disability studies it provides a fulcrum for critique as well. Experiences of embodiment have become a critical nexus that allows scholars to undermine claims to empiricism in the therapeutic and medical sciences. For instance, we recently published an essay with some of our graduate students on "disability as political subjectivity" featuring the exposés of clinical and therapeutic sciences by workers in those fields who later moved over to disability studies (Jarman et al. 2002). This address of impairment is not intended to further entrench bodies as deviant, but rather to illuminate the ways in which disabled bodies and disability-identified researchers provide new perspectives on a mainstream culture greatly affected by medicalized and therapeutic perspectives. As contemporary historians of feral children have shown, the story of Victor and others like him is ultimately one of the institutions in which they found themselves imprisoned.

Yet, in situating disability studies in proximity to the rehabilitation sciences in the contemporary university, disabled students and faculty inevitably find themselves in awkward situations through their interactions with medically based researchers. For instance, when challenged on the belief that all disabilities result in "functional impairments," researchers in the therapies try to reclaim "impairment" as essential to their fields. As one occupational therapist explained: "Impairment is the term used by those who study impairment, so I think it should remain in the terminology without qualification . . . to achieve a balance." It seems that even in the face of exceptions the therapies *will* have their impairments. But the exclusively derogatory connotations of the term have been systematically and rigorously challenged by disability studies. We need to promote a language of adaptation rather than dysfunctionality in order to contest even the most empirical claims. This approach provides more than mere niceties or euphemisms about disability and its attendant material conditions. There is a level of arrogance in the simplistic equation of disability with undesirable deviation; rather than eschew scientific approaches as inherently detrimental, disability studies has to take on these materials on their home disciplinary turf. We recently participated in the production of an *Encyclopedia of Disability* (Albrecht et al. 2005) in which many of the "condition entries" were written by disabled scholars. Those authors did not shy away from the material impact of impairment on their bodies, but they also contextualized their analyses within more involved phenomenological approaches. Thus, one can find an entry on "cerebral palsy" that discusses the difficulties of fine and large motor control, alongside a discussion of the soothing sensation of tremors. If disability studies aims to revolutionize available approaches to human differences, the therapies must challenge and complicate their own one-sided investment in vocabularies of pathology.

The focus on disability as impairment results in tensions when disabled and nondisabled students participate in the same academic program. In several disability studies programs, therapy-based students and faculty have sometimes complained that disabled students make them feel uncomfortable in the classroom because they critique therapies as oppressive to their own sense of self-worth. Such a charge amounts to an argument that the therapies have been unfairly maligned by disabled people, but there is little effort to come to terms with why this perspective is so widely shared by their constituencies. Itard ultimately viewed his experiment with Victor as a failure, not because his subject had failed to master a variety of skills deemed appropriate by the institution, but rather because he never came to appreciate the effort that had been made to "civilize" him. In other words, Victor's lack of reciprocity was the quality found most damning by his rehabilitators.

Disabled students in a disability studies program are much less likely to complete their course of study than are nondisabled students. We attribute the lower rate of completion to the depletion of students' resources because of relatively inaccessible university environments and the demoralization resulting from continuous exposure to the often patronizing ideologies of the "helping professions."

There are two common characteristics of disabled students who have

197

been successful in the program. The first group consists of students who already live near campus so that they have experience negotiating the inaccessibility of their local environments. These individuals represent a population of people who have committed significant resources, time, and energy to the politics of making their local areas accessible. Their political savvy allows them to recognize the obstacles to accessibility on campus as part and parcel of a larger accessibility problem. The second group, surprisingly, consists of what we refer to as *international disability refugees*, those who are fleeing the inhospitality of their home cultures. Often these students have come to disability studies programs with advanced degrees but have come up against an employment "glass ceiling" in their places of origin. Through their frustrations with a lack of disability awareness abroad they arrive already adept at navigating a social environment fraught with difficulties. In other words their initial frustration and intolerance of inclusion failures has already steeled them to the obstacles they encounter on foreign soil.

The difficulties and petty humiliations endured by people with disabilities in the academy are the aftereffects of the fact that universities were set up to exclude disabled people. Historically, disabled people have been objects of study but not purveyors of the knowledge base of disability. Because of the fraught history of the relationship between physical, sensory, and cognitive disabilities, universities as institutions that champion "reason" and "pursuit of the life of the mind" have presumed that disability is an automatic disqualifier from participation. The academy finds itself hard pressed to provide physical access, alternative text/communication strategies, and/or alteration of the pace of its intellectual environment as an accommodation to people with disabilities. Like Victor maneuvering the alien-based terrain of the Institute for Deaf-Mutes, the field of disability studies and its practitioners still find themselves trying to negotiate the most basic necessities toward the meaningful inclusion of disabled people in an environment built to study but not to involve them in its intellectual goals. Consequently, on most campuses a continuum of human variations cannot be translated into an investment in the diversity of thought that such variation represents.

Unwittingly, and perhaps somewhat unwillingly, disability studies has become a crossroads for an international disability community seeking to occupy a shared cultural terrain among likewise stigmatized, yet intellectually minded, individuals. The field needs to recognize the value of this and grow more international in its critique (and less Eurocentric in its models). The future of the field depends upon its ability to take up this challenge in a way that does not replicate the global commodification of other identities.

This entails a thoroughgoing recognition that Western-based methodologies have limited utility for apprehending disability in other cultural contexts. As many scholars in the field now recognize, disability studies is under increasing pressure from globalization to serve as a base for disabled movements and to recognize the degree to which playing that role results from cultural privilege. But one must recognize that the field will be inadequate to the task. The vitality—or anti-institutional "wildness," as we have been calling it—will also spring from a new global traffic in disability issues that can offset early twentieth-century commerce in disparaging eugenic ideologies. We have identified three significant areas where disability studies can sustain and continually reinvigorate its radical potential: (1) through its continuing proximity to, and critique of, the adjustment-based and pathologizing professions; (2) through the active inclusion of activist and arts-based communities to the relevance of its own disciplinary insights; and (3) through its commitment to play self-reflexive host to a growing international disability movement that will inevitably challenge the Western bias of the field.

TEXTS AND PEOPLE-BASED RESEARCH PRACTICES   We conclude with a few cautionary tales addressed to those participating in new efforts to involve disabled people in research on their own experiences. Even in disability studies we are running the risk of reproducing research methodologies that may contribute to the "exhaustion of people-based research practices." As we have argued, research that involves human subjects often replicates the oppressive history of time and energy depletion that is one of the primary sources of disabled people's subjugation. Even in the press to act "morally" and "with the interests of disabled people in mind" within contemporary university settings, we cannot afford to misrecognize the oppressive practices developed out of this history of training and diagnosis applied to feral children, of schooling for blind and deaf individuals, and of the eugenics movement and its effects. All research on disability has been conducted under similar "ethical" precepts—even the most rabid eugenicists argued that their work was performed on behalf of the target population as an alleviation of societal "problems." One can witness disability studies research practices in the social sciences as they marshal in students, community residents, and professionals with disabilities, as if this population were an ever-flowing fount of information. Beneath the guise of "liberal" agendas of disability-identified research practices, the field still reproduces oppression in the name of a "newfound" respect for disabled people's input into the bottomless well of the university's quest for disability knowledge.

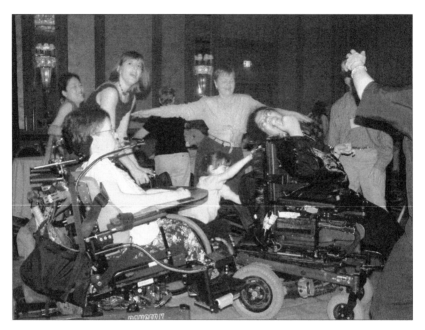

DANCE PARTICIPANTS AT THE ANNUAL SOCIETY FOR DISABILITY
STUDIES CONFERENCE, BETHESDA, MARYLAND, 2003

Further, even in universities where one can spot some leanings toward radical research agendas for disability, one sees an escalating tendency toward methodologies variously called participatory research, client-based research, or community consultation. Contemporary disability studies scholars (and we include ourselves as participants in this research glut) can be found interviewing disabled children about their experiences in schools; holding numerous meetings with people of color in wheelchairs to promote advocacy of their rights; surveying their own students about the transformational aspects of their work in disability studies; bringing in people with Down syndrome to participate in physical exercise programs; performing follow-up interviews with people who have managed releases from nursing homes; comparing the weight of people with developmental disabilities from one decade to another to assess their improving or declining health; or asking families about their frustration with service delivery, inadequate inclusion practices, sibling experiences of growing up with disabled brothers or sisters, and attitudes toward disabled family members. In other words, we do not necessarily see the modern disability research industry concerned with enacting an appropriate level of restraint with respect to the value of disabled people's pursuit of their own objectives. We are running the risk of reproducing aspects of an oppressive structure that disability studies was expected to correct or, at least, avoid.

We end by making a heretical claim that textually based analysis is the only *absolute* remedy to the exhaustion of people-based research practices. First, no matter what its limitations, a study of texts exhausts no one other than the researcher (and, perhaps, the original author). There is a great practicality to approaching disability as an object of study in this manner. Throughout this discussion we have sought to reread the textual record of Victor, the wild boy of Aveyron, as a basis for analyzing the process of institutionalization of disability studies in the contemporary academy. This historical referencing strategy was purposeful in that we believe the existing textual record is more than adequate for current reflections on the "state of disability." There is a need for a radical research-based agenda articulated from this point of view: since texts provide us access to perspectives that inevitably filter disability through the reigning ideologies of their day, their analysis proves tantamount to turning social beliefs into an object of investigation. Just as disability studies has argued vociferously about the socially constructed nature of disability, we must recognize that texts supply windows onto social contexts (including present ones) for our scrutiny.

Because most people have the majority of their interactions with disability through written and visual materials, the analysis of this domain can provide significant interventions into the public representation of bodily, sensory, and cognitive difference. While such an analysis often entails exposing debilitating depictions, this cultural work is necessary and even paramount to influencing the ideological agenda of disability.

In other words, to some extent we have placed the emphasis incorrectly if we value texts only for their "empowering" representations of people with disabilities. We should rest assured that our own era's beliefs about disability will be found wanting in the future, just as the social model is already coming under attack from various quadrants of the disability universe—including disability studies and disability activism. This is one reason why we counsel students against the usage of "positive" and "negative" as adequate terms for assessing the value of visual and/or textual representations. A "positive" image in our time quickly becomes a later moment's insufficiency of portrayal, a barometer by which one assesses that which was overlooked, left out, or depreciated. The ideological moorings of our own era's representational strategies can quickly become dated. Representations are inevitably bound to their own historical moment's shortcomings, idiosyncrasies, and obsessions. Disability studies, like all minority and identity areas of study, must engage all

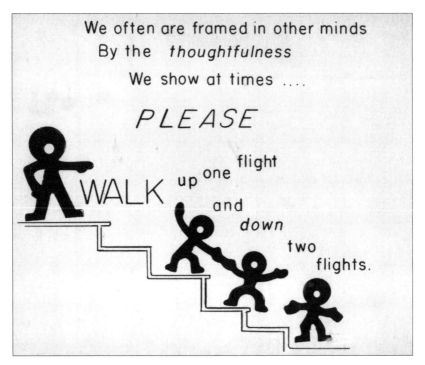

THE MORALITY OF MOBILITY IN INSTITUTIONAL SETTINGS AS SEEN IN A WALL POSTER
FROM THE FORMER INSTITUTION FOR SEVERELY RETARDED AND
CRIPPLED CHILDREN, CHICAGO

images as if they function in the spaces of cultural mediation. One of the primary tasks of disability studies is to cultivate media and textual critics, in the therapies as well as in the humanities, who can intervene in the cultural images of disability that influence our responses and ways of imagining human differences.

This is a pressing issue. Everyone is exposed to such images, even those who are least aware of the glut of disability portrayals that saturate our environment each day. As the media philosopher Michael Ventura (1988) argues: the media are "our most immediate environment" (173). We exist among media as we exist in the air that we breathe; they pervade our atmosphere and we imbibe them without thinking about the involuntary nature of our intake. Disability studies must draw attention to these matters and, in so doing, recognize textual and visual materials as arenas of pragmatic intervention. In assessing representation, we analyze our most immediate environment (as well as the attitudinal environments of those who have gone before us), rather than waiting months, years, or decades for policies to be shaped and implemented or longitudinal demographic studies to be compiled. The interpretation of textual and visual materials delivers objects of intervention that provide an opportunity to reformulate our attitudinal milieu immediately—and in the most pragmatic and visceral manner.

In our perspective, the field of disability studies has functioned most productively as a meta-institutional formation whose primary goal is to destabilize the existing discourses of disability. Its first order of operation, then, is that which exposes the *dependencies* of those fields that would situate disabled people as *dependent*. Victor's dependency on the institution was only made literal once he found himself subject to the regulations of its operations. His life outside was controlled by the demands of the social only to the extent that he found himself forced to forage for his own subsistence (he reportedly raided gardens and trash to supplement his hunting and foraging efforts). Thus, once in Paris there was a good deal of mutual accommodation to be negotiated between Victor as an object of study and those who had traditionally produced the knowledge base that would circumscribe professional and public opinion.

To move from the passive position of the silenced object of discourse in the cultural locations of disability to the active position of producer of knowledge about the social, political, and phenomenological aspects of disability destabilizes any number of objectifying practices. This change alone will prove monumental not because people with disabilities inherently know the truth of their own social and biological lives, but rather because their visible entry into the discourse of their bodies makes all speaking positions in the field shift, becoming necessarily self-conscious and increasingly self-reflexive. Herein lies the source of much of the discomfort posed by disability studies—and also its radical promise.

NOTES

INTRODUCTION

1. Our title alludes to Homi Bhabha's collection of essays on postcolonial theory, *Locations of Culture*. For Bhabha's purposes, the idea of the location of culture pointed toward the underlegitimated locations of resistance or counter-narratives occupied by colonized peoples. While the standard Western reading of culture tended to legitimize only the colonizer's discourse as truly "cultured" or "authentic," Bhabha's reading of colonial texts recognized that those people oppressed by unequal colonial and postcolonial power structures also found opportunities for alternative discourses that competed with dominant cultural production. In seeking to metaphorize the means by which resistant subjects engaged in counter-narrative efforts, Bhabha used the figure of a staircase as an unacknowledged "in-between," where postcolonial populations could maneuver undetected among colonial planes of knowledge: "The stairwell as liminal space, in-between the designators of identity, becomes the process of symbolic interaction, the connective tissue that constructs the difference between upper and lower, black and white. The hither and thither of the stairwell, the temporal movement and passage that it allows, prevents identities at either end of it from settling into primordial polarities. This interstitial passage between fixed identifications opens up the possibility of a cultural hybridity that entertains difference without an assumed or imposed hierarchy" (1994, 4). While this is a compelling analysis of resistance, the unfortunate choice of the stairway as a metaphor for sites of political mobility and insurgency, if literalized, would exclude many subjects (postcolonial and otherwise) with disabilities from actions of resistance. This book seeks a similar analysis that is indebted to Bhabha and other theorists of social power relations. Yet we also seek to identify alternative "spaces" that disabled people occupy as

uniquely marginalized populations. Our resignification of Bhabha's compelling title is purposeful in that the accommodation of disability rights efforts often requires a transformation of political discourse itself.

2. In their essay, "Bodies in Motion: Critical Issues between Disability Studies and Multicultural Studies" (2002), Andrew Jakubowicz and Helen Meekosha argue that the move to multiculturalism is often a new prototypical eugenics in the sense that the bodies that come to represent "minority" groups are often made to be exemplary, noble specimens of ethnicity. The essay goes on to discuss the defeat of efforts at Hunter College in New York City to include disability studies among other courses that fulfill the multicultural curriculum requirement.

3. Readers interested in sites of disability authentication and insider resistance might look at recent disability-related documentary film productions, such as these documentary videos: *Vital Signs: Crip Culture Talks Back* (1995), Billy Golfus's *When Billy Broke His Head* (1995), and *Self Preservation: The Art of Riva Lehrer* (2004). See also recent essays on disability culture (Peters 2000) and "body-based" performance art (Fox 2002; Sandahl 2003; Siebers 2002).

4. See, for example, histories of the Berkeley Independent Living Center and Ed Roberts in Joseph Shapiro's *No Pity* (1994), and the Rolling Quads' claim of rights of access to public locations, such as universities and neighborhoods, in Ruth O'Brien's *Crippled Justice* (2001). Other accounts of disability culture and activist histories in the United States can be found in alternative popular press publications such as *Mainstream Magazine, The Disability Rag, Newsletter on Chronic Illness and Disease, Mouth Magazine, New Mobility Magazine, Ragged Edge,* and *GnarlyBone News,* among others. In addition there are various Web sites devoted to these causes, such as *The Electric Edge* (http://www.ragged-edge-mag.com/), Mothers from Hell 2 (http://www.mothersfromhell2.org/), and Through the Looking Glass (http://www.lookingglass.org/index.php). Finally, more academic analyses of the development of disability cultural and activist communities can be found in works such as Paul Longmore's *Why I Burned My Book* (2003) and Simi Linton's *Claiming Disability* (1998).

5. In numerous ways our own work on disability-based art and representation in *The Body and Physical Difference* (Mitchell and Snyder, eds., 1997) and *Narrative Prosthesis* (2000), as well as other publications in humanities-based disability studies, has sought to reclaim lost or devalued histories of disabled people's perspectives in art, literature, and film. These efforts at historical and arts-based analysis have drawn much of their interpretive momentum from the impetus of cultural and activist efforts to reimagine disability as a socially meaningful experience with its own analytical import. In these approaches humanities scholars seek ways of demonstrating that disability is a socially constructed phenomenon imbued with the values and ideologies of specific historical and cultural moments. They also seek to demonstrate the ways in which disabled people have used a variety of artistic mediums to complicate such perceptions of their bodies.

6. Our own analysis of eugenics is significantly indebted to other disability scholars who have undertaken parallel analyses of eugenics as a formative history in the cultural situation of disabled people today. In particular, we would acknowledge the important work of James Trent, *Inventing the Feeble Mind: A History of Mental Retardation in the United States* (1994); and Anne Kerr and Tom Shakespeare's introduc-

tory text, *Genetic Politics: From Eugenics to Genome* (2002). For a recent analysis of eugenics in relation to modern management systems, see Kliewer and Drake's "Disability, Eugenics, and the Current Ideology of Segregation: A Modern Moral Tale" (1998).

7. Works that theorize modernity as the development of bureaucratic and taxonomic management systems for bodies designated as "nonstandard" include Adorno and Horkheimer 2000; Bauman 2001b; Black 2003; Chesterton and Perry 2000 [1929]; Davis 1995; Ferguson 1994; Fredrickson 2002; Giddens 1991; S. Gilman 1996; Gilroy 2001; Gould 1996 [1981]; Kerr and Shakespeare 2002; Ordover 2003; Pernick 1996; Ronell 1989; Stone 1984; and Stiker 1999.

8. The recent publication of Foucault's lectures from the early 1970s (Foucault 2003) provides an important case in point. Foucault traces out a developed history of the movement from categories of monstrosity to the invention of medically verifiable diagnostic pathologies during the nineteenth century. "Monstrosity" is a classification situated largely outside of human adjudication, while designations of "abnormal" are increasingly taken up by pathologizing professions, such as psychiatry. Abnormal subjects can be "treated" and managed within research and confinement system, while monsters prove more liminal to human comprehension tactics. Thus, disability can be recognized as a category that continues to resonate with a now archaic conception of monstrosity, while also existing in the domain of empirical pathology.

9. Histories of UPIAS are widely available. See the University of Leeds Web-based archive for some primary source documents produced between 1974 and 1983 by this organization: http://www.leeds.ac.uk/disability-studies/archiveuk/UPIAS/UPIAS.htm.

10. For instance, Galton (2001 [1869]) argues that in colonial Africa "it may prove that the Negroes, one and all, will fail as completely under the new conditions [British colonialism] as they have failed under the old ones, to submit to the needs of a superior civilization to their own; in this case their races, numerous and prolific as they are, will in course of time be supplanted and replaced by their betters" (40). Likewise in the case of women, Galton dismissively argues that his study only needs to account for male genius because "still less consistent with decorum would it have been, to introduce the names of female relatives that stand in the same category" (47). Finally, with respect to Native Americans, the author explains that in the times of Indian attacks "great [European] men of eminence" became "heroes of their own situation" for "they were cool in danger, sensible in council, cheerful under prolonged suffering, humane to the wounded and sick, encouragers of the faint hearted" (87). Never does it occur to Galton that the expression of "eminence" might be embodied in the military tactics of the colonized or in the council of their female leaders. Galton had to dismiss social advantage as a byproduct of class, culture, and education in order to correlate biology with destiny—particularly in the case of race and feeblemindedness, as the two classifications that he used most consistently to cross-reference each other. It was not an accident that no women or people of color populated his list of "geniuses" in history, but rather that superior heredity was seen as responsible for the degree of one's social recognition (95–369).

11. We initially made this argument about the use of disability in liberationist discourse in the introduction to our edited collection titled *The Body and Physical Difference: Discourses of Disability*: "while disability, at first glance, would seem to share with other socially stigmatized identities visible physical characteristics that link

external or perceptible differences to internal deficits, critical parallels with other minoritized identities have been slow in coming. . . . Indeed, the push to expose physical difference as an ideological phantasm has, ironically, resulted in the further reification of disability as the term absented from our social models" (Mitchell and Snyder, eds., 1997, 5).

12. Many societies repeat habits of shame concerning physical and biological outcasts, though the exact features of the bodies involved may differ. For instance, one consistently finds, across cultures and geographies, families that exhibit shame about their disabled members, and the widespread cultural recognition of this leads to globalized oppressive practices. At the same time, many cultures participate in stories of heroic overcoming that further entrench (rather than alleviate) social disapprobation. Yet this social narrative remains largely reserved for family associates and cultural caregivers who can be held responsible by social majorities for putting up with the "burden" of disabled people. As a result, disability studies exposes how these stories are ultimately disadvantageous to disabled subjects themselves. Or rather, if the actions of disabled individuals are cited as the source of overcoming, then it is only to the extent that they successfully distance themselves from the stigma of their own biologies. In either case, debilitating narratives of disability, whether as shameful existence or personal overcoming stories, usually function as *secondhand* accounts of disability told by those who place distance between themselves and disabled people.

These secondhand social narratives form the foundation of widespread cultural policing practices around disabled bodies. They are also the impetus for crafting restrictive disability policy at national and local levels. They constitute the social domain for the cultivation of increasingly severe management, confinement, and degradation practices. They are the back-and-forth schemes that constitute a discourse of disability and a dialectic about disabled persons that, most significantly, keeps the disabled body limited to a select role—as informant, lab rat, recipient, token exemplar of progress, and nowadays the liberated consumer of assistive technologies and *social* (instead of *medical*) interventions.

13. Labels, in these scenarios, serve more as indicators of a social situation than as empirical descriptions of literal bodily or cognitive topographies. In this we would depart from Hacking, who has argued that the natural sciences produce analyses of "indifferent kinds," while the social sciences and humanities attend to "interactive kinds." Our readings suggest that often disabled people confront efforts in the biological and rehabilitation sciences to turn "interactive kinds" into "indifferent kinds" (that is, objects without meaningful cognizance of their classification type). For disability studies and body studies scholars, it is important to refuse the presumed universality that disability labels acquire when referring to dynamic human conditions.

CHAPTER ONE

1. In *The Discovery of the Asylum* David Rothman (1971) argues that debates about public responsibility for those who were ill or incapacitated during the seventeenth and eighteenth centuries largely revolved around questions of looking out for one's own members. Disability and poverty did not turn a person into an outcast. Families and communities were expected to provide support for those who could not support themselves. Most poverty discussions developed around the definition of member-

ship in order to release communities from having to support nomads and paupers who might migrate into the settlement.

2. In " 'Too Much of a Cripple' " (Mitchell and Snyder 1999) we argue that Ishmael ends up aborting his initial efforts to apply the sciences of physiognomy and phrenology to the interpretation of the whale. After demonstrating that these sciences of the visible have nothing to contribute to the understanding of the whale, Ishmael brushes them off as "semi-sciences" (Melville 1993 [1850], 345) that "like every other human science is but a passing fable" (347). The novelist's return to these subjects in *The Confidence-Man* helps to demonstrate the influence such practices continued to have on nineteenth-century interpretive practices. Because disabled people were viewed as possessing bodily and cognitive deviances that expressed the corruption of their souls, they were particularly at risk for dehumanizing treatment produced by the analysis of appearances.

3. By looking at disability as a cultural effort to fix a field of sliding signifiers into an exclusively derogatory identity, one may gain a glimpse of *The Confidence-Man's* overarching rhetorical strategy. Just as the confidence game can be played from multiple social vantage points—corporate executive, paralyzed black pauper, vacationing stockbroker, one-legged customs officer, snake-oil salesman, and giant—the body's myriad meanings also prove indeterminate. Efforts to identify an accord between physical presentation and internal motivation place Melville's work squarely within the context of nineteenth-century physiognomic thinking. Although physiognomy has a lengthy social history, it came to be consolidated as an empirical science in the late eighteenth century following the publication of Swiss theologian Johann Caspar Lavater's efforts to catalogue facial countenances into reliable personality types. For Lavater, physical features functioned as symptomatic expressions of internal dispositions, and thus the external body could be considered a means of grasping the otherwise intangible truth of an individual's moral character. As a technique of interpretation developed before the invention of instruments that allowed medical practitioners to "see" into the body (such as the stethoscope, microscope, and x-ray), physiognomy promoted the body as a reliable textual system to be "read" by trained professionals and amateurs alike.

4. This shift in the representation of disability may be accounted for in a variety of ways, but many biographers have remarked upon the "serious illness" that Melville experienced between the writing of *Moby-Dick* and *The Confidence-Man*. His back problems worsened and he endured a debilitating bout of sciatica in 1855, his eyesight grew increasingly untrustworthy, and he was bedridden for a significant period as a result. It was during this time that Melville's family also began to worry over his sanity. Yet, while most critics have attempted to attribute the dark vision of *The Confidence-Man* to these bodily "afflictions," we would argue that Melville's body forced him to interrogate his own ideas of ability. The sea change that takes place between 1850 and 1857 may have placed disability as a maligned social identity on a par with race in the author's mind, and thus the story becomes a vehicle for exploring this new relationship in the way that racial relations would be probed in *Moby-Dick*.

5. Both Henri-Jacques Stiker's *History of Disability* (1999) and Jean Starobinski's *Largesse* (1997) explore the rise of charity networks overseen by the Catholic Church in the Middle Ages. Charity, according to both theorists, sets into motion a social hierarchy of relations that are both economic and religious in nature. The object of

charity, social "unfortunates" such as disabled people and single women with children, are situated in an objectifying position where their maintenance benefits the social order and the religious prospects of the upper classes. Within such an analysis charity does not "lift up" the unfortunate, but rather enthralls them to a system that maintains a position of subordination. Thus, a system that presumably works in the name of poor and disabled people (overdetermined by other marked characteristics, such as gender, race, sexuality, and ability) functions to further disenfranchise them by turning them into managed populations. The object of charity must surrender everything except membership in the category of the "deserving poor."

6. Winthrop offers charity as a form of good works, even though Puritanism followed strict Calvinistic teachings in rhetorically rejecting this concept as a route to redemption. According to Puritan teachings, God had already predetermined who would be saved, and thus, one could not *earn* one's way to salvation through the performance of beneficent deeds. Yet charitable acts continued to function as one of the key signs of individual election, because those predestined for heaven would inevitably practice good works as an outgrowth of their divinely anointed standing.

7. Thus, the mercantilist moorings of Winthrop's rhetoric become apparent. As a relatively wealthy lawyer, Winthrop formulates economics and religion as parallel systems. The contract of citizens among themselves to support and sustain each other, and also with God who will watch over them as long as they pursue a properly Christian life, serves as the crossover covenant. Like a loan between consenting parties sealed through a binding contract, charity would seal an agreement to which parishioners and God would commit. Thus, the Puritans formulated their religious and economic relations along the same rhetorical lines.

8. In her article "Hawthorne's Reconceptualization of Transcendentalist Charity," Monika Elbert (1997) cites Yates's report on the poor from 1824 as arguing that " 'men of great literary acquirements . . . have insisted, that distress and poverty multiply in proportion to the funds created to relieve them, and that the establishment of any poor rates is not only unnecessary, but hurtful' (949). But Yates also pointed out the undue cruelty imposed upon the poor, the isolation of the poor as if they were felons, and the shortcomings of the economic system in providing jobs for the poor (951–952)" (2).

9. Serres (1982b) borrows the term *parasite* from information theory to identify what he calls a logic of interruption that keeps systems of communication from becoming static and singular. The parasite is a principle of fluidity where "noise"—that which upsets pure communication from reaching its destiny without adulteration—feeds upon a system seeking to homogenize and force data into a stable commodity. Thus, while the term *parasite* has many hues of negative value—distortion, chaos, disruption, interruption, nonproducer, and so forth—Serres performs an operation that would liberate parasitism into a desirable and necessary value. Yet this theory of the "in-between" as the space of the parasite is not entirely romanticized as the place of possibility. As systems seek to monopolize and dominate disorder, they do so through a function of scapegoating. Following on the heels of theorist René Girard, Serres's scapegoat becomes a primary preoccupation of systems—scapegoating is another name for the activity of exclusion where the parasite is suppressed in order to give orderliness primacy. As Steven D. Brown explains with respect to the scapegoat

function in Serres's work: "the social bond arises as an attempt to thwart a primal violence of all-against-all. Such violence can only be tamed when it is re-directed towards a particular individual—the scapegoat—upon whom the massed violence of the crowd falls" (2002, 8). Thus, while the parasite becomes the condition of possibility for systems as they pursue their drive toward homogeneity and stasis, the exclusion of chaotic creativity made possible by the parasite proves the foundation of social violence. As the parasite is sought out and excluded, the collective avoids exacting violence upon itself (the violence of all against all) through a displacement onto a singular representative that occupies the site of incoherence and irrationality. One of the astonishing attributes in Serres's descriptions of systems and their operations with respect to the parasite is the language of disability from which so many of his theories derive. Not only does the vocabulary of parasite, accommodation, mutation, and deviation hail from communications theory, such terms are also central to disability studies and the historical construction of disabled people. If disability is characterized as a difference that cannot be sufficiently accommodated within the social body, then Serres's theory of the parasite can prove productive for theories of disability as well (one could argue, however, that disability is the ever-present excluded term in Serres's own theoretical system).

10. In his essay "Considerations by the Way" Emerson (1982) lays out his argument against charity in the following fashion: "The worst of charity is, that the lives you are asked to preserve are not worth preserving. Masses! the calamity is the masses. I do not wish any mass at all, but honest men only, lovely, sweet, accomplished women only, and no shovel-handed, narrow-brained, gin-drinking million stockingers or lazzaroni at all" (1081). Thoreau's attack on philanthropists occurs in "Economy" (1973): "The philanthropist too often surrounds mankind with the remembrance of his own cast-off griefs as an atmosphere, and calls it sympathy" (121); while in "Life without Principle" (1998 [1863]) he argues: "To be supported by the charity of friends, or a government pension . . . is to go into the almshouse" (160).

11. While the quick fix functions as the primary interaction in the first half of *The Confidence-Man*, a more tortuous discursive structure characterizes the second half of the work. Once the Cosmopolitan enters the scene, the discourse on charity increasingly appears in the guise of oral tales exchanged among the passengers. In these oral monologues, brutal stories of social injustice, such as John Moredock's Indian hating, Charlemont's sudden turn to madness, and China Aster's failed business acumen, all subject the characters in question to debasing social myths of biologically based inferiority. Thus, physical disability becomes aligned with race and madness as marked social bodies. These anecdotes imported into the direct economic encounters on board the *Fidèle* expand the repertoire of social conditions that condemn one to a form of embodiment. In addition, such stories serve to disrupt the overall narrative flow of *The Confidence-Man* by providing diversions that move the listener/reader out of the immediate environment. These diversions introduce what Serres would call static into the overarching narrative system. They function as textual deviations about the meaning of deviance itself and, in doing so, participate in the performative structure of a work that tries to "embody" the concepts it seeks to articulate.

12. In *Melville's Anatomies*, Otter (1999) carefully details the development of craniometry and phrenology in the nineteenth-century United States as a backdrop for

Melville's critique of reliance on the visible as an empirical practice. In our essay " 'Too Much of a Cripple' " (1999), we provide a similar analysis of Melville's critique of physiognomy. In both cases Melville's later works are situated as a challenge to the professionalizing empirical sciences of his time.

CHAPTER TWO

1. The main tenets of disability studies center on efforts to forward human differences as part of a continuum of human biology. Such an approach displaces pathologies as the guiding medical paradigm and installs a social model that recognizes and celebrates physical and cognitive variations as integral to human existence.

2. In *The Body in Pain*, Elaine Scarry (1985) argues that a phenomenon that manifests itself on the "face of the Earth" receives the validity of a visual representation. Pain often lacks visible markers, since it occurs within the subject, so its validity is often disputed or held with suspicion. In sequestering citizens with disabilities, eugenics effectively sought to eradicate certain degrees of human difference from the visible cultural record. One might theorize that hiding disability from view seeks to perform a scientific sleight-of-hand. The extraction of people with disabilities from the social mainstream curtails any need to accommodate a range of human differences. In espousing this objective, the culture misplaces efforts to support those with disabilities in favor of eliminating certain human types.

3. This phrase is adopted from Steven Noll's (1995) book, *Feeble-Minded in Our Midst*, which focuses upon the treatment of those with "mental retardation" in the South since the eugenics period.

4. On social Darwinism, see Bannister (1979), who argues that the conceptualization of Darwinian "survival of the fittest" proved a bastardization of adaptive principles. Instead, the theory evolved from a misconceived conjoining of the theories of Spencer and Darwin. The originary eugenics work of Sir Francis Galton helped to popularize this misreading, and many eugenicists went on to repeat the formulation, which contributed to its acceptance in public and professional circles. On the restrictive nature of anti-immigration laws as they pertain to disabled people, see Baynton 2001. On charity, see our discussion in chapter 1 of Winthrop's sermon, "A Modell of Christian Charity," delivered off the shores of New England.

5. In our book *Narrative Prosthesis: Disability and the Dependencies of Discourse* (Mitchell and Snyder 2000), we analyze the work on disability by the sixteenth-century French philosopher Michel de Montaigne. Particularly in his essay, "Of a Double-Bodied Child," Montaigne (1971b) argues that disability is not a sign of divine disfavor but rather an example of "the infinities of forms that evidence the diversity of God's work."

6. In spite of the usual arguments about the benefits of pastoral settings to feeble-minded individuals, Goddard also argued the opposite: "Fifty years ago the problem was not as serious as it is today, because these defectives were out in the world by themselves, getting killed by a runaway horse, or falling into machinery, or in some way meeting an untimely death. Today we are exceedingly careful; we are protecting them in every possible way; we are taking care of them in our institutions and giving them every advantage, and then sending them out into the world—a menace to the rest of humanity" (1916, 8). Such contradictory rationale shows the extent to which eugenics researchers would go to rationalize the incapacities of their subjects.

CHAPTER THREE

1. This neglect of the violence committed by the state against disabled people has resulted in serious consequences. In the *Garrett* case, the U.S. Supreme Court ruled against the applicability of the Americans with Disabilities Act to two Alabama employees who had lost their jobs due to the onset of disability. In this instance, the majority opinion, written by Justice Brennan, argued that "the ADA's legislative record fails to show that Congress identified a history and pattern of irrational employment discrimination by the States against the disabled." Although the record did include catalogues of abuses, Chief Justice Rehnquist wrote that "the great majority of these incidents do not deal with state activities in employment" (Amici Curiae 2000). Since eugenics was developed as an argument about disabled people's inability to work in an increasingly competitive industrial economy, the entire movement could be described as a "history and pattern of irrational employment discrimination by the States against [disabled people]."

2. The Enlightenment is the historical period responsible for the initial constitution of "disability" as the designation of human variation as inferiority. While pre-Enlightenment forms of discrimination occurred primarily with respect to religious practices and cultural customs that were deemed alien, European empirical practices gave increasing momentum to biology as the appropriate locale of deviation. Thus, while leper colonies and institutions for blind or deaf people existed in the Middle Ages, species distinctions invested with hierarchies of value gained momentum as a means of determining desirable human characteristics. For instance, Francis Bacon's essays from the early 1500s distinguish between beauty and deformity as divergent embodiments where desirability is accorded solely to the former category. As empirical science was bolstered by methodologies such as taxonomies, statistics, measurement, heredity, genetics, and IQ testing, human bodies and cognition came to be assessed primarily with respect to characteristics identified as normative.

3. As a further indicator of the instability of the social construction of Jewishness an opposing theory of genetic threat also surfaces in modernity. Lennard Davis has pointed out to us that even if Jews didn't assimilate (or rarely did) in a genetic sense, the threat was their ability to assimilate culturally and economically (personal communication, 6 January 2003). The danger was also configured as the Jew's "race" (i.e., peculiar hereditary essence) infiltrating the realms of power, culture, and finance, while maintaining at least a fantasy of cultural purity. Such an assimilationist threat was attributed to feebleminded "carriers" as well, who were believed to pass on their tainted qualities without overt manifestation of the "symptoms" of inferiority. Thus, their reproduction could proceed unchecked by scientific and state management schemes promoted by eugenicists.

4. U.S. eugenicists such as Howe were fond of disparaging the tendency of the French school to foreground the positive characteristics of their institutional charges when describing their "idiocy": "Besides, when [Séguin] is giving descriptions of individual idiots, to illustrate his subject, he always places their manifestations of intelligence in the foreground of the picture" (Howe 1848, 18). This practice apparently threatened to undermine eugenics practices by giving too much credit to its custodial objects!

5. In coining the term *eugenics*, the British researcher Sir Francis Galton sought to challenge the Darwinian theory of undirected gradualist evolution by organisms.

Through the establishment of deterministic hereditary patterns, Galton argued, it would be possible to intervene in Nature by selective breeding among humans as well as plants and animals for desirable characteristics. In formulating the theory of the polyhedron, Galton, according to Stephen Jay Gould (2002, 348), tried to overturn the radicality of Darwin's recognition that lack of intentionality governed the evolutionary process, by adopting a principle of homogeneity as the banal rule of Nature. Thus, for Galton, human variations represented by congenital disabilities proved undesirable and out of accord with all organisms' penchant for stasis and the reproduction of sameness. Yet Gould's massive study overlooks eugenic theories as borrowing from saltationist discourses of evolution and, in doing so, uncritically enshrines Galton's work as progressive for its time.

6. Efforts to undermine the humanity of disabled people continue along this pseudo-empirical route of argumentation. For instance, Princeton professor Peter Singer promotes the argument that some disabled children should be passively euthanized because they lack the sentience that his brand of utilitarianism accords to fully "human" organisms. Such arguments characterized nearly all eugenic sentiments; they hinge upon scientific and philosophical willingness to empty certain individuals of qualities and thus reduce them to a state of mere matter. In the section titled "The Negro Is Only Biological," Gilroy convincingly argues that such a rhetorical tactic has also been used historically against blacks: "These black bodies are no longer to be supervised by the souls that were once imagined to outlive them. There are no souls here; they have been banished by the fatal affirmation of carnal and corporeal vitality" (2001, 255).

CHAPTER FOUR

1. Our comparison of Wiseman with Foucault is intended to draw parallels between visual and textual methodologies. Rather than claim Wiseman as a student of Foucault, our argument places these two figures alongside each other. Since both began their work in the 1960s, they lived through an era that was marked by civil rights activism—particularly the vocal anti-institutionalization movement. This shared social milieu was the backdrop to their work.

2. In our essay, "Out of the Ashes of Eugenics" (Snyder and Mitchell 2002), we argue that the eugenicist category of "the feebleminded" included an expansive array of disabilities. In this sense eugenics provided the first "modern" grouping of disability as a variety of inferior classifications based upon biological variation. We argue that individuals labeled with cognitive, sensory, or physical disabilities are more intertwined in each other's fates than has been traditionally recognized.

3. Patriarchal colonial authority consistently linked the birth of disabled children with the blasphemies of women who sought to challenge male religious and civil authority. Consider, for instance, the expulsion of the antinomian heretic Ann Hutchinson from Massachusetts to Rhode Island. Shortly after her banishment, Hutchinson was rumored to have given birth to a "monstrous child" as further sign of her corruption (Hall 1991, 17).

4. Humanitarian missions to incarcerate people with disabilities in institutions have often been premised on cure or intervention. As in the case of the Helen Keller Institute in Wiseman's films, the promise of imminent return to the community based upon successful treatment ultimately fails to materialize to any significant extent, and

the institution quickly becomes a full-time custodial structure. We refer to this historical movement from rehabilitation to custodianship in institutions as the operation of a "diagnostic regime" (Snyder and Mitchell 2002). In doing so, we seek to identify a pattern or overriding "logic" of modern institutionalization.

5. The theory of a "body" made to speak the truth of the state can also be found in Scarry's work (1985). In her analysis, torture becomes a tool of the state as it attempts to coerce the body into confirming a regime's authority and interpretive mastery.

6. Material on Frederick Wiseman's documentary Web site (www.zipporah.com) quotes reviewers extolling the humanity and tolerance of institutional and administrative personnel. For instance, a reviewer, John J. O'Connor, writing in the *New York Times*, comments that "the interracial harmony of the school is a model for all institutions. And the devotion and skills of the staff are positively inspiring."

CHAPTER FIVE

1. The probing of psychic identifications in film criticism has produced a significant body of work: Teresa De Lauretis's *Technologies of Gender: Essays on Theory, Film, and Fiction* (1987) and *Alice Doesn't: Feminism, Semiotics, Cinema* (1984); Linda Williams's "Film Bodies: Gender, Genre, and Excess" (1999); Vivian Sobchack's *Address of the Eye: A Phenomenology of Film Experience* (1991); and William Paul's *Laughing Screaming: Modern Hollywood Horror and Comedy* (1994); among many others.

2. For a critical assessment of this strategy of identifying positive and negative stereotypes of disability in visual media, see our analysis in *Narrative Prosthesis: Disability and the Dependencies of Discourse* (Mitchell and Snyder 2000, 17–21).

CHAPTER SIX

1. Several studies have helped revive the significance of feral children to Western traditions of inquiry: Harlan Lane's *Wild Boy of Aveyron* (1979); Roger Shattuck's *Forbidden Experiment: The Story of the Wild Boy of Aveyron* (1980); and Michael Newton's *Savage Girls and Wild Boys: A History of Feral Children* (2003). We draw our comparison between the institutional status of disability studies and these authors' analyses of feral children as objects of exhibition and remediation.

2. Foucault underscores the use of disabled people's anatomies as a baseline for understanding the general population's "health" in *The Birth of the Clinic* (1975). In exchange for "donated healthcare" the medical industry used the bodies of disabled, ill, racialized, and lower-class people to help improve the treatment of those who could afford medical attention. This point was also made by Rebecca Maskos in our documentary *A World without Bodies* (2002), when she ironically pointed out that the bodies of murdered disabled victims during the Holocaust were allowed to serve as referents for "normal" bodies while failing to be considered "human" at the same time.

3. As we discuss in chapter 3, Michael Newton (2003) retells the stories of seven feral children captured in Europe, Asia, the United States, India, Africa, and Russia between 1800 and the late twentieth century. The cases show how various human differences are treated as animal-like and socially deviant; in each case we witness individuals subject to scientific investigation against their will.

4. For instance, Spivak describes the colonial mission in terms of efforts to per-

petually scrutinize native differences: "The archival, historiographic, disciplinary-critical, and, inevitably, interventionist work involved here is indeed a task of 'measuring silence.' This can be a description of 'investigating, identifying, and measuring . . . the *deviation*' from an ideal that is irreducibly different" (1988, 286–87). Similarly, Homi Bhabha explains the process of differentiation as an effect of power: "The exercise of colonial authority, however, requires the production of differentiations, individuations, identity effects through which discriminatory practices can map out subject populations" (1994, 111). In each case the production of subjugated identities becomes an effect of a power that would—as in the case of disability—produce ceaseless degrees of difference. This production of differences, in turn, allows the knowledge-producing culture to pose as a transparent, coherent, and whole subject. We analyze the seemingly infinite array of deviations that characterize disability in medicine and rehabilitation as a product of a similar discriminatory and discriminating mode of authority.

5. In *The History of Disability*, Henri-Jacques Stiker (1999) analyzes René Girard's anthropological model of scapegoating as expressions of violence toward disabled people. For Girard via Stiker, communal punishment toward people with deformities or disabilities surfaces out of desires for mimesis: "human desire is mimetic; it seeks to appropriate the desire and the objects of another. The crisis that is the consequence can be resolved only by the ritual sacrifice of a victim, a scapegoat that makes it possible to expel the violence and leave the possibility of a livable communal space. This victim mechanism not only deflects violence (although always only temporarily) but also conceals it" (30).

WORKS CITED

Note: Many of the primary sources utilized in this study are archived in the Smith Ely Jelliffe Eugenics Collection, nine privately bound volumes, in the personal library of David Braddock, University of Colorado, Boulder. Citations to documents in this collection are as complete as the collection allows. The collection is cited throughout as "Smith Ely Jelliffe Eugenics Collection."

Abbot, E. Stanley. 1919. "Preventable Forms of Mental Disease and How to Prevent Them." *Massachusetts Society for Mental Hygiene* 12:1–28. Reprinted from *Boston Medical and Surgical Journal* 97, no. 16 (20 April 1916): 555–63. Smith Ely Jelliffe Eugenics Collection.

Adorno, Theodor. 1994. "Messages in a Bottle." In *Mapping Ideology*, ed. S. Žižek, 34–45. London: Verso.

Adorno, T., and M. Horkheimer. 2000. "Elements of Antisemitism." In *Theories of Race and Racism: A Reader*, ed. L. Back and J. Solomos, 206–11. New York: Routledge.

Albrecht, G., J. Bickenbach, D. Mitchell, W. Schalick, and S. Snyder, eds. 2005. *Encyclopedia of Disability*. 5 vols. Thousand Oaks, Calif.: Sage Publishing.

Aly, G., P. Chroust, and C. Pross, eds. 1994. *Cleansing the Fatherland: Nazi Medicine and Racial Hygiene*. Baltimore: Johns Hopkins University Press.

Amici Curiae. 2000. Document filed on behalf of over a hundred historians, to ensure that evidence of widespread state discrimination against persons with disabilities is not forgotten. U.S. Supreme Court, *Garrett v. Board of Trustees of the University of Alabama*, October term, 2000. http://www.bazelon.org/alabamabrief .html (accessed 21 April 2001; no longer available).

Anderson, V. V. 1919. *Mental Defect in a Southern State: Report of the Georgia Commission on Feeblemindedness and the Survey of the National Committee for Mental Hygiene.* New York: National Committee for Mental Hygiene. 28 pp. Reprinted from *Mental Hygience* 3, no. 4: 527–65.

Annas, George J., and Michael A. Grodin, eds. 1992. *The Nazi Doctors and the Nuremberg Code: Human Rights in Human Experimentation.* New York: Oxford University Press.

Atkins, Thomas R., ed. 1976. *Frederick Wiseman.* New York: Monarch.

Atwood, Charles Edwin. 1907. "The School Training of Backward Children in the New York Public City Public Schools." New York: A. R. Elliott Publishing Co. 10 pp. Reprinted from *New York Medical Journal,* 7 September. Read before the Medical Society of the County of New York, 27 May 1907, as part of a symposium on mental defectives. Smith Ely Jelliffe Eugenics Collection.

Audet, G. 1923. "The Vermeylen Method for the Detection of Mental Deficiency: The Psychographic Examination of Intelligence." 39 pp. Smith Ely Jelliffe Eugenics Collection.

Back, Les, and John Solomos. 2000. "Introduction: Theorizing Race and Racism." In *Theories of Race and Racism: A Reader,* ed. L. Back and J. Solomos, 1–32. New York: Routledge.

Bailey, Pearce. N.d. "Backward and Defective Children." New York State Commission for Mental Defectives. 26 pp. Smith Ely Jelliffe Eugenics Collection.

Baizley, Doris, and Victoria Ann Lewis. 1997. "Selected Scenes from: 'P.H.*reaks: The Hidden History of People with Disabilities.'" In *Staring Back: The Disability Experience from the Inside Out,* ed. Kenny Fries, 303–32. New York: Plume Books.

Baldwin, Bird T. N.d. "The Psychology of Mental Deficiency." *Popular Science Monthly,* 82–93. Smith Ely Jelliffe Eugenics Collection.

Bannister, Robert C. 1979. *Social Darwinism: Science and Myth in Anglo-American Social Thought.* Philadelphia: Temple University Press.

Barnes, Colin. 1996. "The Social Model of Disability: Myths and Misrepresentations." *Coalition,* August, 27–33.

———. 1999. "Disability Studies: New or Not So New Directions?" *Disability and Society* 14, no. 4: 577–80.

———. 2003. "What a Difference a Decade Makes: Reflections on Doing 'Emancipatory' Disability Research." *Disability and Society* 18, no. 1: 3–17.

Bauman, Zygmunt. 2001a. *The Individualized Society.* Cambridge: Polity Press.

———. 2001b. *Modernity and the Holocaust.* Ithaca, N.Y.: Cornell University Press.

Baynton, Doug. 2001. "Defectives in the Land." In *The New Disability History: American Perspectives,* ed. P. Longmore and L. Umansky, 1–16. New York: New York University Press.

Berger, John. 1995. *Ways of Seeing.* New York: Viking.

Bernstein, Charles. 1920. "Colony and the Extra-Institutional Care for the Feebleminded." Reprinted from *Mental Hygiene* 4, no. 1 (January): 1–28. Smith Ely Jelliffe Eugenics Collection.

Berry, Richard J. A, and S. D. Porteus. 1918. "A Practical Method for the Early Recognition of Feeble-Mindedness and Other Forms of Social Inefficiency." *Training School Bulletin* 15, no. 6 (whole number 158): 81–92. Smith Ely Jelliffe Eugenics Collection.

Bess, Thomas. 1930. "Mental Defectives and Sterilization." 20 pp. Reprinted from *West Virginia Medical Journal* 26, no. 4 (April). Read before the Kanawha Medical Society, Charleston, West Virginia, 7 January 1930. Smith Ely Jelliffe Eugenics Collection.

Bhabha, Homi. 1994. *Locations of Culture*. New York: Routledge.

Black, Edwin. 2003. *War against the Weak: Eugenics and America's Campaign to Create a Master Race*. New York: Four Walls Eight Windows.

Blake, Mabelle B. 1917. "The Defective Girl Who Is Immoral." *Boston Medical and Surgical Journal* 177, no. 14 (4 October): 492–94. Read before the Conference on Feeble-mindedness of the Massachusetts Society for Mental Hygiene, Boston, 14 December 1916. Smith Ely Jelliffe Eugenics Collection.

Bragg, Lois. 1997. "From the Mute God to the Lesser God: Disability in Medieval Celtic and Old Norse Literature." *Disability and Society* 12, no. 2: 165–77.

British Medical Association. 1932. *Report of the Mental Deficiency Committee*. "As presented to the Annual Representative Meeting of the Association, 1932, and ordered by the Council of the Association to be published." London: British Medical Association. Smith Ely Jelliffe Eugenics Collection.

Brown, Eleanor Gertrude. 1934. *Milton's Blindness*. New York: Columbia University Press.

Brown, Steven D. 2002. "Michel Serres: Myth, Mediation and the Logic of the Parasite." http://devpsy.lboro.ac.uk/psygroup/sb/Serres.htm (accessed 14 February 2004; no longer available).

Browne, Dennis. 1966. "The Problem of Byron's Lameness." *Proceedings of the Royal Society of Medicine*.

Burleigh, Michael. 1994. *Death and Deliverance: "Euthanasia" in Germany, 1900–1945*. Cambridge: Cambridge University Press.

Butler, Judith. 1993. *Bodies That Matter: On the Discursive Limits of "Sex."* New York: Routledge.

———. 1999. *Gender Trouble: Feminism and the Subversion of Identity*. New York: Routledge.

Byrom, Brad. 2001. "A Pupil and a Patient: Hospital Schools in Progressive America." In *The New Disability History*, ed. P. Longmore and L. Umansky, 133–56. New York: New York University Press.

Byron, Lord George. 1901. *The Works of Lord Byron: Poetry, Vol. 5*, ed. E. H. Coleridge, 467–534. New York: Charles Scribner's Sons.

———. 1905. *The Deformed Transformed*. In *The Poetical Works of Lord Byron*, ed. Ernest Hartley Coleridge, 722–44. London: John Murray.

Canguilhem, Georges. 1991. *The Normal and the Pathological*. New York: Zone Books.

Carlson, Elof Axel. 2001. *The Unfit: A History of a Bad Idea*. Cold Spring Harbor, N.Y.: Cold Spring Harbor Laboratory Press.

Carlson, Licia. 2001. "Cognitive Ableism and Disability Studies: Feminist Reflections on the History of Mental Retardation." *Hypatia* 16, no. 4: 124–46.

Carstens, C. C. 1917. "What It Means to Have Non-Committed Feeble-Minded in the Community." *Boston Medical and Surgical Journal* 177, no. 14 (4 October): 486–89. Smith Ely Jelliffe Eugenics Collection.

Chambers, Ross. 1991. *Room for Maneuver: Reading (the) Oppositional (in) Narrative*. Chicago: University of Chicago Press.

Chesterton, G. K., and M. Perry. 2000 [1929]. *Eugenics and Other Evils: An Argument against the Scientifically Organized State.* Seattle, Wash.: Inkling Books.

Clare, Eli. 1999. *Exile and Pride.* New York: Consortium.

Clark, L. Pierce, and Charles E. Atwood. 1922. "A Contribution to the Etiology of Feeblemindedness with Special Reference to Prenatal Enamel Defects." *New York Medical Journal and Medical Record,* 17 May, 1–25. Smith Ely Jelliffe Eugenics Collection.

Clarkson, R. D. 1920. "Care of Mentally Defective Children." *Journal of Psycho-Asthenics* 26 (June 1920–June 1921): 375–82. Smith Ely Jelliffe Eugenics Collection.

Clell, Madison. 1998. *Cuckoo: One Woman's True Stories of Living with Multiple Personality Disorder.* Madison, Wis.: Green Door Studios.

Cliff, Michelle. 1988. "A Journey into Speech." In *Multi Cultural Literacy,* ed. R. Simmonson and S. Walker. St. Paul, Minn.: Graywolf Press.

Cobb, O. H. 1925. "Educating and Placing Out Mental Defectives." Reprinted from *Journal of the Iowa State Medical Society* 15 (March): 1–4. Read at the annual meeting of the Medical Society of the State of New York, Rochester, 22 April 1924. Smith Ely Jelliffe Eugenics Collection.

Coleridge, Peter. 1993. *Disability Liberation and Development.* Oxford: Oxfam.

Conway, Catherine E. 1917. "Report of Mental Examination of Thirty-Seven Children Ten Months after the First Examination." State Board of Charities: Mental Examinations, No. 9. *Eugenics and Social Welfare Bulletin* (Albany, N.Y.): 42–59. Smith Ely Jelliffe Eugenics Collection.

Coriat, Isador H. 1915. "Some New Symptoms in Amaurotic Family Idiocy." *Boston Medical and Surgical Journal,* 1 July, 20–21. Smith Ely Jelliffe Eugenics Collection.

Corker, Mairian. 1999. "Differences, Conflations, and Foundations: The Limits to 'Accurate' Theoretical Representation of Disabled People's Experience?" *Disability and Society* 14, no. 5: 71–76.

Cowie, Elizabeth. 1999. "The Spectacle of Actuality." In *Collecting Visible Evidence,* ed. J. Gaines and M. Renov, 19–45. Minneapolis: University of Minnesota Press.

Cravens, Hamilton. 1988. *The Triumph of Evolution: The Heredity-Environment Controversy, 1900–1941.* Baltimore: Johns Hopkins University Press.

Crow, Liz. 1996. "Including All of Our Lives: Renewing the Social Model of Disability." In *Encounters with Strangers: Feminism and Disability,* ed. J. Morris, 206–26. London: Women's Press.

cummings, e. e. 1980 [1926]. *Complete Poems 1913–1962.* New York: Harcourt Brace Jovanovich.

Darden, O. B. 1912. "Reports on Defective Children: Mental Defectives, the Anemic, the Tuberculous, the Blind, the Deaf and Dumb, the Crippled." Report presented to the Virginia Board of Education, 11 December 1912. Smith Ely Jelliffe Eugenics Collection.

———. 1932. "Moral Subnormality as an Expression of Mental Unsoundness." Reprinted from *Virginia Medical Monthly,* March, 1–12. Read by invitation before the Fourth District Medical Society, Rocky Mount, North Carolina, 10 November 1931. Smith Ely Jelliffe Eugenics Collection.

Darwin, Charles. 1997 [1871]. *Descent of Man and Selection in Relation to Sex.* Buffalo, N.Y.: Prometheus Books.

———. 1998 [1859]. *On the Origin of Species.* New York: Gramercy.

Davis, Lennard. 1995. *Enforcing Normalcy: Disability, Deafness, and the Body.* New York: Verso.

———. 2002. *Bending Over Backwards: Essays on Disability and the Body.* New York: New York University Press.

De Lauretis, Teresa. 1984. *Alice Doesn't: Feminism, Semiotics, Cinema.* Bloomington: Indiana University Press.

———. 1987. *Technologies of Gender: Essays on Theory, Film, and Fiction.* Bloomington: Indiana University Press.

Desrosiers, Alain. 2002. *The Politics of Large Numbers: A History of Statistical Reasoning.* Cambridge, Mass.: Harvard University Press.

Deutsch, Helen. 1996. *Resemblance and Disgrace: Alexander Pope and the Deformation of Culture.* Cambridge, Mass.: Harvard University Press.

Deutsch, Helen, and Felicity Nussbaum, eds. 2000. *"Defects": Engendering the Modern Body.* Ann Arbor: University of Michigan Press.

Dick, Alex. 2000. "Poverty, Charity, Poetry: The Unproductive Labors of 'The Old Cumberland Beggar.'" *Studies in Romanticism* 39, no. 3: 365–96.

Dillingham, William B. 1986. *Melville's Later Novels.* Athens: University of Georgia Press.

Doll, E. A. 1916a. "Note on the 'Intelligence Quotient.'" *Training School Bulletin* (Vineland, N.J.) 7 (January): 1–6. Smith Ely Jelliffe Eugenics Collection.

———. 1916b. "Preliminary Note on the Diagnosis of Potential Feeble-Mindedness." Reprinted from *Training School Bulletin* (Vineland, N.J.) 13 (June): 1–8. Read at the San Francisco meeting of the American Psychological Association, 5 August 1915, under title "Diagnostic Value of the Binet Tests." Smith Ely Jelliffe Eugenics Collection.

———. 1917. *Clinical Studies in Feeble-Mindedness.* Boston: Gorham Press.

Drewry, William Francis. 1912. "The Mental Defectives." *Virginia Medical Semi-Monthly,* 26 January, 1–21. Read in part before the Southside Virginia Medical Association, Lawrenceville, December 1911. Smith Ely Jelliffe Eugenics Collection.

Dunn, Katherine. 2002 [1983]. *Geek Love.* New York: Vintage.

Edson, Andrew W. 1912. "The Education and Training of Feebleminded Children in the Public Schools." *New York Medical Journal,* 7 December, 1176–78. Smith Ely Jelliffe Eugenics Collection.

Elbert, Monika. 1997. "Hawthorne's Reconceptualization of Transcendentalist Charity." *ATQ: The American Transcendentalist Quarterly* 11, no. 3: 213–32.

Emerson, Ralph Waldo. 1981. "Nature." In *The Portable Emerson,* 7–50. New York: Penguin Books.

———. 1982. "Consideration by the Way." In *Emerson in His Journals,* ed. Joel Porte. Cambridge, Mass.: Belknap Press of Harvard University Press.

Epstein, Julia. 1995. *Altered Conditions: Disease, Medicine, and Storytelling.* New York: Routledge.

Farrell, Elizabeth. 1912. "Subnormality." Smith Ely Jelliffe Eugenics Collection.

Ferguson, Phil. 1994. *Abandoned to Their Fate: Social Policy and Practice toward Severely Retarded People in America, 1820–1920*. Philadelphia: Temple University Press.

Fernald, Walter. 1893. "The History of the Treatment of the Feebleminded." In *Proceedings of the National Conference of Charities and Correction*, 203–21. Boston: Press of George H. Ellis.

———. 1912. "The Burden of Feeble-Mindedness." *Journal of Psycho-Asthenics* 17, no. 3: 87–111. Delivered as the Annual Discourse before the Massachusetts Medical Society, 12 June 1912. Smith Ely Jelliffe Eugenics Collection.

———. 1914. "The Diagnosis of the Higher Grades of Mental Defect." Reprinted from *American Journal of Insanity* 70, no. 3 (January): 253–64. Smith Ely Jelliffe Eugenics Collection.

———. 1915. "What Is Practicable in the Way of Prevention of Mental Defect." Massachusetts Society for Mental Hygiene. 8 pp. Reprinted from *Proceedings of the Conference Committee on State Care of the Insane, Feeble-minded and Epileptic*. Read before the National Conference of Charities and Correction, Baltimore, 1915. Smith Ely Jelliffe Eugenics Collection.

Finger, Anne. 1997. "Helen and Frida." In *Staring Back: The Disability Experience from the Inside Out*, ed. Kenny Fries, 255–63. New York: Plume Books.

Finkelstein, Vic. 1996. "Outside, 'Inside Out.'" *Coalition*, April, 30–36.

Fitts, Ada M. 1916. "How to Fill the Gap between Special Classes for Mentally Defective Children and Institutions." Massachusetts Society for Mental Hygiene. No. 21: 1–8. Reprinted from *Ungraded* 2, no. 1 (October). Read before the National Conference of Charities and Corrections, Indianapolis, May 1916. Smith Ely Jelliffe Eugenics Collection.

Foner, Eric. 1995. *Free Soil, Free Labor, Free Men: The Ideology of the Republican Party before the Civil War*. New York: Oxford University Press.

Foucault, Michel. 1975. *The Birth of the Clinic: An Archaeology of Medical Perception*. New York: Vintage Books.

———. 1988a. *The Care of the Self: The History of Sexuality, Vol. 3*. New York: Pantheon Books.

———. 1988b. *Madness and Civilization: A History of Insanity in the Age of Reason*. New York: Vintage Books.

———. 1994. *Order of Things: An Archaeology of the Human Sciences*. New York: Vintage Books.

———. 1995. *Discipline and Punish: The Birth of the Prison*. New York: Penguin Books.

———. 1997. "Psychiatric Power." In *Ethics: Essential Works of Foucault, 1954–1984*, ed. Paul Rabinow, 39–50. New York: New Press.

———. 2000a. "The Politics of Health in the Eighteenth Century." In *Power: Essential Works of Foucault, 1954–1984*, ed. Paul Rabinow, 90–105. New York: New Press.

———. 2000b. "The Punitive Society." In *Power: Essential Works of Foucault, 1954–1984*, ed. Paul Rabinow, 23–38. New York: New Press.

———. 2003. *Abnormal: Lectures at the Collège de France*. New York: Picador.

Fox, Ann M. 2002. "Res(crip)ting Feminist Theater through Disability Theater: Selections from the Disability Project." *NWSA Journal* 14, no. 3: 99–119.

Fox-Keller, Evelyn. 1996. *Refiguring Life*. New York: Columbia University Press.

Fraser, Kate. N.d. "Feeble-minded Children: An Inquiry into Mental Deficiency in School-Children, with Special Reference to Syphilis as a Causative Factor, as Determined by the Wassermann Reaction." *School Hygiene*, 100–107. Smith Ely Jelliffe Eugenics Collection.

Fredrickson, George. 2002. *Racism: A Short History*. Princeton, N.J.: Princeton University Press.

Freeman, R. Austin. 1923. "The Sub-Man." *Eugenics Review*, July, n.p. Smith Ely Jelliffe Eugenics Collection.

French, Sally. 1994. "What Is Disability?" In *On Equal Terms: Working with Disabled People*, ed. Sally French, 3–16. Oxford: Butterworth Heinemann.

Friedlander, Henry. 1997. *The Origins of Nazi Genocide: From Euthanasia to the Final Solution*. Chapel Hill: University of North Carolina Press.

Friedlander, Saul. 1997. *Nazi Germany and the Jews: The Years of Persecution, 1933–1939*. New York: Harper Collins.

Gallagher, Hugh. 1989. *By Trust Betrayed: Patients, Physicians, and the License to Kill in the Third Reich*. New York: Henry Holt.

Galton, Francis. 1988 [1889]. *Natural Inheritance*. New York: AMS Press.

———. 2001 [1869]. *Hereditary Genius: An Inquiry into Its Laws and Consequences*. Honolulu: University Press of the Pacific.

Gelb, Stephen. 2002. "Charles Darwin's (Mis)use of Intellectual Disabilities in *The Descent of Man*." Presented at annual meeting of Society for Disability Studies, Washington, D.C., 2003.

Gerber, David. 2000. *Disabled Veterans in History*. Ann Arbor: University of Michigan Press.

Giddens, Anthony. 1991. *The Consequences of Modernity*. Stanford, Calif.: Stanford University Press.

Gilman, Charlotte Perkins. 1998 [1898]. *Women and Economics: A Study of the Economic Relation between Women and Men*. Mineola, N.Y.: Dover.

Gilman, Sander. 1985. *Difference and Pathology: Stereotypes of Sexuality, Race, and Madness*. Ithaca, N.Y.: Cornell University Press.

———. 1996. *Seeing the Insane*. Lincoln: University of Nebraska Press.

Gilroy, Paul. 1995. *The Black Atlantic: Modernity and Double Consciousness*. Cambridge, Mass.: Harvard University Press.

———. 2001. *Against Race: Imagining Political Culture across the Color Line*. Cambridge, Mass.: Harvard University Press.

Gleeson, Brendan. 2001. "Domestic Space and Disability in Nineteenth-Century Melbourne, Australia." *Journal of Historical Geography* 27, no. 2: 223–40.

Glueck, Bernard. 1913. "The Mentally Defective Immigrant." National Committee of Mental Hygiene Reprint No. 9. New York: A. R. Elliot Publishing Co. 22 pp. Reprinted from *New York Medical Journal*, 18 October. Smith Ely Jelliffe Eugenics Collection.

Goddard, Henry H. 1910a. "Heredity of Feeble-Mindedness." *American Breeders Magazine* 1, no. 3: 165–78. Smith Ely Jelliffe Eugenics Collection.

———. 1910b. "A Measuring Scale of Intelligence." Vol. 6, no. 11 (whole number 71): 3–11. Smith Ely Jelliffe Eugenics Collection.

———. 1911. "The Elimination of Feeble-Mindedness." *Annals of the American*

Academy of Political and Social Science, March, 505–16. Smith Ely Jelliffe Eugenics Collection.

———. 1914. *Feeble-Mindedness: Its Causes and Consequences*. New York: Macmillan.

———. 1915. *The Criminal Imbecile: An Analysis of Three Remarkable Murder Cases*. New York: Macmillan.

———. 1916. "The Menace of Mental Deficiency from the Standpoint of Heredity." *Boston Medical and Surgical Journal* 175, no. 8 (24 August): 269–71. Read before the conference of the Massachusetts Society for Mental Hygiene, Boston, 19 November 1915. Smith Ely Jelliffe Eugenics Collection.

———. 1918. "The Possibilities of Mental Hygiene in Cases of Arrested Mental Development." *Training School Bulletin* 15, no. 6: 67–72. Presented at the Tenth Congress of the American School Hygiene Association, Albany, New York. Smith Ely Jelliffe Eugenics Collection.

———. 1973 [1912]. *The Kallikak Family: A Study in the Heredity of Feeble-Mindedness*. New York: Arno Press.

Goffman, Erving. 1961. *Asylums: Essays on the Social Situation of Mental Patients and Other Inmates*. New York: Doubleday.

———. 1986. *Stigma: Notes toward the Management of Spoiled Identity*. New York: Simon and Schuster.

Gould, George M., and Walter L. Pyle. 1901. *Anomalies and Curiosities of Medicine: Being An Encyclopedic Collection of Rare and Extraordinary Cases, and of the Most Striking Instances of Abnormality in All Branches of Medicine and Surgery, Derived from an Exhaustive Research of Medical Literature from Its Origin to the Present Day, Abstracted, Classified, Annotated and Indexed*. London: W. B. Saunders.

Gould, Stephen Jay. 1996 [1981]. *The Mismeasure of Man*. Expanded edition. New York: Norton.

———. 2002. *The Structure of Evolutionary Theory*. Cambridge, Mass.: Belknap Press of Harvard University Press.

Griggs, B. 2003. "Dual Status of Disability, Race Studies." *Salt Lake Tribune*, 3 October.

Grosskurth, Phyllis. 1997. *Byron: The Flawed Angel*. New York: Houghton Mifflin.

Haberman, J. Victor. 1918. "A Psychopathic Constitution Resembling So-Called Moral Insanity, and Its Interpretation." *Boston Medical and Surgical Journal* 178, no. 6 (7 February): 194–96. Smith Ely Jelliffe Eugenics Collection.

Hacking, Ian. 1990. *The Taming of Chance*. New York: Cambridge University Press.

———. 2000. *The Social Construction of What*. Cambridge, Mass.: Harvard University Press.

Hall, David. 1991. *Witch-hunting in Seventeenth Century New England: A Documentary History, 1638–1692*. Boston: Northeastern University Press.

Harley, Harrison L. 1916. "Some Observations on the Operation of the Illinois Commitment Law for the Feebleminded." *Chicago Medical Recorder*, 350–51. Smith Ely Jelliffe Eugenics Collection.

Harris, Benjamin. 1671. *The Fables of Young Aesop, with Their Morals: With a Moral History of His Life and Death, Illustrated with Forty Curious Cuts Applicable to Each Fable*. London: Benjamin Harris.

Hastings, George A. N.d. [c. 1917]. "Some Essentials of a State Program for Mental Hygiene." New York: Committee on Mental Hygiene, State Charities Aid Association. Pp. 3–14. Smith Ely Jelliffe Eugenics Collection.

Heine, Helme. 1989. *The Marvelous Journey through the Night*. Translated by Ralph Manheim. New York: Farrar, Straus, and Giroux.

Hickson, W. J. 1914. "Organic Brain Lesions in Mental Defectives." *Illinois Medical Journal* 26:394–400. Smith Ely Jelliffe Eugenics Collection.

Holmes, Martha Stoddard. 2003. *Fictions of Affliction: Physical Disability in Victorian Culture*. Ann Arbor: University of Michigan Press.

Howe, Samuel Gridley. 1848. *Report Made to the Legislature of Massachusetts upon Idiocy*. Boston: Coolidge and Wiley.

Huet, Marie-Hélène. 1998. *Monstrous Imagination*. Cambridge, Mass.: Harvard University Press.

Hughes, Bill, and Kevin Paterson. 1997. "The Social Model of Disability and the Disappearing Body: Towards a Sociology of Impairment." *Disability and Society* 12, no. 3: 325–40.

Ireland, William W. 1898. *The Mental Affections of Children, Idiocy, Imbecility and Insanity*. London: J. and A. Churchill.

Irwin, Elizabeth A. 1913. "A Study of the Feeble-Minded in a West Side School in New York City." *Training School Bulletin* 10, no. 5 (September): 65–76. Smith Ely Jelliffe Eugenics Collection.

Jakubowicz, Andrew, and Helen Meekosha. 2002. "Bodies in Motion: Critical Issues between Disability Studies and Multicultural Studies." *Journal of Intercultural Studies* 23, no. 3: 237–51.

Jarman, Michelle, et al. 2002. "Theorizing Disability as Political Subjectivity: Work by the UIC Disability Collective on Political Subjectivities." *Disability and Society* 17, no. 5: 555–69.

Johnson, Mary. 2003. *Make Them Go Away: Clint Eastwood, Christopher Reeve and the Case against Disability Rights*. New York: Avocado Press.

Jones, Douglas Lamar. 1984. "The Transformation of the Poverty Law in Eighteenth-Century Massachusetts." In *Law in Colonial Massachusetts, 1630–1900*, ed. Frederick S. Allis Jr., 153–90. Boston: Colonial Society of Massachusetts.

Katz, Michael. 1986. *In the Shadow of the Poorhouse: A Social History of Welfare in America*. New York: Basic Books.

Keith, Lois. 2001. *Take Up Thy Bed and Walk: Death, Disability, and Cure in Classic Fiction for Girls*. London: Women's Press.

Kelso, Robert W. 1917. "Feeble-Mindedness as an Element in Poverty." *Boston Medical and Surgical Journal*, 4 October, 484–87. Read before the Conference on Feeble-mindedness of the Massachusetts Society for Mental Hygiene, Boston, 15 December 1916. Smith Ely Jelliffe Eugenics Collection.

Kerr, Anne, and Tom Shakespeare. 2002. *Genetic Politics: From Eugenics to Genome*. Cheltenham, U.K.: New Clarion Press.

Kesey, Ken. 1962. *One Flew over the Cuckoo's Nest*. New York: Viking Press.

Kevles, Daniel. 1995. *In the Name of Eugenics: Genetics and the Uses of Human Heredity*. Cambridge, Mass.: Harvard University Press.

Kliewer, Christopher, and Stephen Drake. 1998. "Disability, Eugenics and the Current Ideology of Segregation: A Modern Moral Tale." *Disability and Society* 13, no. 1: 95–111.

Knox, Howard A. 1913. "A Test for Adult Imbeciles and Six Year Old Normals." *New York Medical Journal*, 22 November, 1017–18. Smith Ely Jelliffe Eugenics Collection.

Kuhl, Stefan. 1994. *The Nazi Connection: Eugenics, American Racism, and German National Socialism*. New York: Oxford University Press.

Kuhlman, Susan. 1973. *Knave, Fool, and Genius: The Confidence-Man as He Appears in Nineteenth-Century American Fiction*. Chapel Hill: University of North Carolina Press.

Laclau, Ernesto, and Chantal Mouffe. 1984. *Hegemony and Socialist Strategy: Towards a Radical Democratic Politics*. London: Verso.

Lane, Harlan. 1979. *Wild Boy of Aveyron*. Cambridge, Mass.: Harvard University Press.

Langan, C. 2001. "Mobility Disability." *Public Culture* 13, no. 3 (Fall): 459–84.

Lapon, Lenny. 1986. *Mass Murderers in White Coats: Psychiatric Genocide in Nazi Germany and the United States*. Springfield, Mass.: Psychiatric Genocide Research Institute.

Laughlin, Harry H. 1922. *Eugenical Sterilization in the United States: A Report of the Psychopathic Laboratory of the Municipal Court of Chicago*. Chicago: Municipal Court.

Lee, Harper. 1960. *To Kill a Mockingbird*. Philadelphia: J. B. Lippincott.

Liceto, Fortunio. 1634. *De monstrorum natura caussis*.

Lifton, R. 2000. *The Nazi Doctors: Medical Killing and the Psychology of Genocide*. New York: Basic Books.

Limon, John. 1990. *The Place of Fiction in the Time of Science: A Disciplinary History of American Writing*. New York: Cambridge University Press.

Lincoln, David F. 1902. "The Education of the Feeble-minded in the United States." In *Education Report, 1902*, chap. 47, 2157–97. Smith Ely Jelliffe Eugenics Collection.

Linton, Simi. 1998. *Claiming Disability: Knowledge and Identity*. New York: New York University Press.

Longmore, Paul. 1986. "Screening Stereotypes." In *Images of the Disabled/Disabling Images*, ed. A. Gartner and T. Joe, 65–78. New York: Praeger.

———. 1997. "Conspicuous Contribution and American Cultural Dilemmas: Telethon Rituals of Cleansing and Renewal." In *The Body and Physical Difference: Discourses of Disability*, ed. D. Mitchell and S. Snyder, 134–60. Ann Arbor: University of Michigan Press.

———. 2003. *Why I Burned My Book and Other Essays on Disability*. Philadelphia: Temple University Press.

Longmore, Paul, and David Goldberger. 2000. "The League of the Physically Handicapped and the Great Depression: A Case Study in the New Disability History." *Journal of American History* 87, no. 3 (December): 288–322.

Longmore, Paul, and Laurie Umansky. 2001. *The New Disability History: American Perspectives*. New York: New York University Press.

Mack, Maynard. 1985. *Alexander Pope: A Life*. New York: W. W. Norton.

Macy, Mary Sutton. 1913. "The Borderline Case." *Woman's Medical Journal*, February. Read before the Emma Willard Association, New York, 8 January 1913. Smith Ely Jelliffe Eugenics Collection.

Mairs, Nancy. 1998. *Waist-High in the World: Life among the Non-Disabled.* Boston: Beacon Press.

Martin, Douglas. 1997. "Disability Culture: Eager to Bite the Hands That Would Feed Them." *New York Times,* 1 June. http://barrier-free.arch.gatech.edu/Articles/nyt_doll.html (accessed 6 February 2004).

Marx, Karl. 1906. *Capital: A Critique of Political Economy.* Chicago: Charles H. Kerr.

McBroom, D. E. 1923. "Feeble-Mindedness." Reprinted from *Minnesota Medicine,* November, 636–43. Read before the Southern Minnesota Medical Association, Faribault, Minnesota, 11 June 1923. Smith Ely Jelliffe Eugenics Collection.

McFarland-Icke, Bronwyn Rebekah. 1999. *Nurses in Nazi Germany: Moral Choices in History.* Princeton, N.J.: Princeton University Press.

McLuhan, Marshall. 1964. *Understanding Media: The Extensions of Man.* New York: Signet.

McRuer, Robert. 2003. "As Good As It Gets: Queer Theory and Critical Disability." *GLQ: A Journal of Lesbian and Gay Studies* 9, no. 1: 79–105.

Meekosha, H. 1999. "Superchicks, Clones, Cyborgs, and Cripples: Cinema and Messages of Bodily Transformation." *Social Alternatives* 18, no. 1 (Summer).

Melville, Herman. 1984 [1857]. *The Confidence-Man: His Masquerade.* Evanston, Ill.: Northwestern University Press and Newberry Library.

———. 1993 [1850]. *Moby-Dick; or, The Whale.* Evanston, Ill.: Northwestern University Press and Newberry Library.

Michalko, Rod. 2002. *The Difference That Disability Makes.* Philadelphia: Temple University Press.

Miller, Donald S., and Ethel H. Davis. 1969. "Shakespeare and Orthopedics." *Surgery, Gynecology and Obstetrics,* February, 358–66.

Mitchell, David, and Sharon Snyder. 1997. "Introduction: Disability and the Double Bind of Representation." In *The Body and Physical Difference: Discourses of Disability,* ed. D. Mitchell and S. Snyder, 1–21. Ann Arbor: University of Michigan Press.

———. 1999. "'Too Much of a Cripple': Ahab, Dire Bodies, and the Language of Prosthesis in *Moby Dick.*" *Leviathan* 1, no. 1: 5–22.

———. 2000. *Narrative Prosthesis: Disability and the Dependencies of Discourse.* Ann Arbor: University of Michigan Press.

Mitchell, David, and Sharon Snyder, eds. 1997. *The Body and Physical Difference: Discourses of Disability.* Ann Arbor: University of Michigan Press.

Monroe, W. S. 1897. "Feeble-Minded Children in the Public Schools." In *Proceedings of the National Conference of Charities and Corrections,* 5 January, 430–33. Westfield, Mass. Smith Ely Jelliffe Eugenics Collection.

Montaigne, Michel de. 1971a. "Of Cripples." In *The Complete Works of Montaigne: Essays, Travel Journals, Letters,* edited and translated by Donald Frame, 784–91. Stanford, Calif.: Stanford University Press.

———. 1971b. "Of a Double-Bodied Child." In *The Complete Works of Montaigne: Essays, Travel Journals, Letters,* edited and translated by Donald Frame, 538–39. Stanford, Calif.: Stanford University Press.

Morris, Jenny. 2001. "Impairment and Disability: Constructing an Ethics of Care That Promotes Human Rights." *Hypatia* 16, no. 4 (Fall): 1–16.

Morrison, T. 1989. "Unspeakable Things Unspoken: The Afro-American Presence in American Literature." *Michigan Quarterly Review* 28, no. 1: 1–34.

Mosse, G. 2000. "The Jews: Myth and Counter-Myth." In *Theories of Race and Racism: A Reader*, ed. L. Back and J. Solomos, 195–205. New York: Routledge.

Mueller-Hill, Benno. 1988. *Murderous Science: Elimination by Scientific Selection of Jews, Gypsies, and Others, Germany 1933–1945.* Oxford: Oxford University Press.

Nash, Alice M., and S. D. Porteus. 1919. "The Educational Treatment of Defectives." Study No. 3–1919 Series. Vineland, N.J.: Research Laboratory, 1–19. Reprinted from *Training School Bulletin* 18 (November). Smith Ely Jelliffe Eugenics Collection.

Nelkin, Dorothy. 1995. *Selling Science: How the Press Covers Science and Technology.* New York: W. H. Freeman.

Newton, Michael. 2003. *Savage Girls and Wild Boys: A History of Feral Children.* London: Faber and Faber.

Noll, Steven. 1995. *Feeble-Minded in Our Midst: Institutions for the Mentally Retarded in the South, 1900–1940.* Chapel Hill: University of North Carolina Press.

Nussbaum, Felicity A. 1997. "Feminotopias: The Pleasures of 'Deformity' in Mid-Eighteenth-Century England." In *The Body and Physical Difference: Discourses of Disability*, ed. D. Mitchell and S. Snyder, 161–73. Ann Arbor: University of Michigan Press.

O'Brien, Ruth. 2001. *Crippled Justice: The History of Modern Disability Policy in the Workplace.* Chicago: University of Chicago Press.

Oliver, Michael. 1983. *Social Work with Disabled People.* Basingstoke, U.K.: Macmillan.

———. 1990. *The Politics of Disablement.* London: Macmillan.

———. 1996. *Understanding Disability: From Theory to Practice.* New York: St. Martin's Press.

Ordahl, George. 1919. "Industrial Efficiency of the Moron." *Training School Bulletin*, February, 145–59. Smith Ely Jelliffe Eugenics Collection.

Ordover, Nancy. 2003. *American Eugenics: Race, Queer Anatomy, and the Science of Nationalism.* Minneapolis: University of Minnesota Press.

Otter, Samuel. 1999. *Melville's Anatomies.* Berkeley: University of California Press.

Paré, Ambroise. 1982. *Monsters and Marvels.* Chicago: University of Chicago Press.

Paterson, Kevin, and Bill Hughes. 1999. "Disability Studies and Phenomenology: The Carnal Politics of Everyday Life." *Disability and Society* 14, no. 5: 597–610.

Paul, Diane B. 1995. *Controlling Human Heredity: 1865 to the Present.* New York: Humanity Books.

Paul, William. 1994. *Laughing Screaming: Modern Hollywood Horror and Comedy.* New York: Columbia University Press.

Paulson, William R. 1988. *The Noise of Culture: Literary Texts in a World of Information.* Ithaca, N.Y.: Cornell University Press.

Pernick, Martin S. 1996. *The Black Stork: Eugenics and the Death of "Defective" Babies in American Medicine and Motion Pictures since 1915.* New York: Oxford University Press.

———. 1997. "Defining the Defective: Eugenics, Aesthetics, and Mass Culture in Early-Twentieth-Century America." In *The Body and Physical Difference: Discourses of Disability*, ed. D. Mitchell and S. Snyder, 89–110. Ann Arbor: University of Michigan Press.

Peters, Susan. 2000. "Is There a Disability Culture? A Syncretisation of Three Possible World Views." *Disability and Society* 15, no. 4: 583–601.

Peterson, Anna M., and E. A. Doll. 1914. "Sensory Discrimination in Normal and Feeble Minded Children: An Experimental Study of Discrimination of Lifted Weights in Relation to Mental Age." Publications of the Training School at Vineland, New Jersey, Department of Research, No. 3 (December). Vineland, N.J.: Training School. 18 pp. Smith Ely Jelliffe Eugenics Collection.

Peterson, Haynes. 1898. "Idiocy, Imbecility, and Feeble-Mindedness." 663–82. Smith Ely Jelliffe Eugenics Collection.

Pfeiffer, David. 1994. "Eugenics and Disability Discrimination." *Disability and Society* 9, no. 4: 481–99.

———. 2000. "The Devils Are in the Details: The ICIDH2 and the Disability Movement." *Disability and Society* 15, no. 7: 1079–82.

Pickens, Donald K. 1968. *Eugenics and the Progressives*. Nashville, Tenn.: Vanderbilt University Press.

Pickersgill, Joshua. 1803. *The Three Brothers*. 4 vols. London: John Stockdale.

Pollock, Horatio M., and Edith M. Furbush. 1919. *Annual Census of the Insane, Feebleminded, Epileptics and Inebriates in Institutions in the United States, January 1, 1918*, 1–30. New York: National Committee for Mental Hygiene. Reprinted from *Mental Hygiene* 3, no. 1 (January): 78–107. Smith Ely Jelliffe Eugenics Collection.

Possek, R. N.d. "The Causes, Prevention, and Treatment of Visual Defects in School-children." 108–18. Presented at the Seventeenth International Congress of Medicine: Section—Hygiene and Preventive Medicine. Smith Ely Jelliffe Eugenics Collection.

Potter, Howard W. 1922. "Endocrine Imbalance and Mental Deficiency." Detroit, Mich. 20 pp. Reprinted from *Journal of Nervous and Mental Disease* 56, no. 4 (15 June): 334–45. Smith Ely Jelliffe Eugenics Collection.

———. 1923. "The Clinical Organization of the State Institution for Mental Defectives." 2–19. Smith Ely Jelliffe Eugenics Collection.

Proctor, Robert. 1988. *Racial Hygiene: Medicine under the Nazis*. Cambridge, Mass.: Harvard University Press.

Pross, Christian. 1994. *Cleansing the Fatherland: Nazi Medicine and Racial Hygiene*. Baltimore: Johns Hopkins University Press.

Rafler, Nicole Hahn, ed. 1988. *White Trash: The Eugenic Family Studies, 1877–1919*. Boston: Northeastern University Press.

Reilly, Philip R. 1991. *The Surgical Solution: A History of Involuntary Sterilization in the United States*. Baltimore: Johns Hopkins University Press.

Rodgers, Daniel T. 1998. *Atlantic Crossings: Social Politics in a Progressive Age*. Cambridge, Mass.: Belknap Press of Harvard University Press.

Ronell, Avital. 1989. *The Telephone Book: Technology, Schizophrenia, Electric Speech*. Lincoln: University of Nebraska Press.

Rosanoff, Aaron J. 1931. "Sex-Linked Inheritance in Mental Deficiency." 289–97 (September). Smith Ely Jelliffe Eugenics Collection.

Rothman, David J. 1971. *The Discovery of the Asylum: Social Order and Disorder in the New Republic*. Boston: Little, Brown.

———. 1980. *Conscience and Convenience: The Asylum and Its Alternatives in Progressive America*. Boston: Little, Brown.

Rubin, Rita. 2000. "A New Course: Disability Pride—Fight for Rights Sparks New Field of College Study." *USA Today*, 25 July, D1–2.

Ryan, Susan. 2000. "Misgivings: Melville, Race, and the Ambiguities of Benevolence." *American Literary History* 12, no. 4: 685–712.

Sajous, D. E. de M. 1916. "Our Duty to Mental Defectives of the Present Generation." *New York Medical Journal* 103, no. 14 (April): 625–31. Address read by invitation before the New York Polyclinic Clinical Society, 7 February 1916. Smith Ely Jelliffe Eugenics Collection.

Salmon, Dr. 1912. "Immigration and the Admixture of Races in Relation to the Mental Health of the Nation." In *Modern Treatment of Mental and Nervous Diseases*, ed. White and S. E. Jelliffe. Philadelphia. Smith Ely Jelliffe Eugenics Collection.

Samuels, Ellen. 2005. "From Melville to Eddie Murphy: The Disability Con in American Literature and Film." *Leviathan: A Journal of Melville Studies*, forthcoming.

Sandahl, Carrie. 2003. "Queering the Crip or Cripping the Queer? Intersections of Queer and Crip Identities in Solo Autobiographical Performance." *GLQ: A Journal of Lesbian and Gay Studies* 9, no. 1: 25–56.

Sandel, Michael J. 1996. *Democracy's Discontent: America in Search of a Public Philosophy*. Cambridge, Mass.: Harvard University Press.

Sandy, William C. 1932. "The Mental Defective and His Needs." Bureau of Mental Health, Pennsylvania Department of Welfare, Harrisburg. 8 pp. Reprinted from *Pennsylvania Medical Journal*, February. Smith Ely Jelliffe Eugenics Collection.

Scarry, Elaine. 1985. *The Body in Pain: The Making and Unmaking of the World*. New York: Oxford University Press.

Schlapp, M. G. 1918. *Theoretical Considerations of Mental Deficiency*. New York: William Wood.

Schlapp, M. G., and Alice E. Paulsen. 1918. "Report on 10,000 Cases from the Clearing House for Mental Defectives." 11–12. Reprinted from *Medical Record*, 16 February. Smith Ely Jelliffe Eugenics Collection.

Schneider, William. 1982. "Toward the Improvement of the Human Race: The History of Eugenics in France." *Journal of Modern History* 54, no. 2 (June): 268–91.

————. 2002. *Quality and Quantity: The Quest for Biological Regeneration in 20th Century France*. Cambridge: Cambridge University Press.

Schriempf, Alexa. 2001. "(Re)fusing the Amputated Body: An Interactionist Bridge for Feminism and Disability." *Hypatia* 16, no. 4 (Fall): 53–79.

Searcy, J. T. N.d. "Heredity: An Allegory." In *Insane and Epileptic: Report of Committee*, 286–303. Tuscaloosa, Ala. Smith Ely Jelliffe Eugenics Collection.

Serres, Michel. 1982a. *Hermes: Literature, Science, Philosophy*. Edited by J. V. Harari and D. F. Bell. Baltimore: Johns Hopkins University Press.

————. 1982b. *The Parasite*. Baltimore: Johns Hopkins University Press.

Shakespeare, Tom. 1994. "Cultural Representation of Disabled People: Dustbins for Disavowal." *Disability and Society* 9, no. 3: 283–99.

————. 1997. "Defending the Social Model." *Disability and Society* 12, no. 2: 293–300.

Shakespeare, Tom, and Tom Watson. 1995. "Habeamus Corpus? Sociology of the Body and the Issue of Impairment." Paper presented at Quinquennial Aberdeen University Conference.

Shapiro, Joseph. 1994. *No Pity: People with Disabilities Forging a New Civil Rights Movement*. New York: Three Rivers Press.

Shattuck, Roger. 1980. *The Forbidden Experiment: The Story of the Wild Boy of Aveyron*. London: Quartet Books.

Shaw, Barrett. 1994. *The Ragged Edge: The Disability Experience from the Pages of the First Fifteen Years of The Disability Rag*. Louisville, Ky.: Avocado Press.

Sherry, M. 2000. "Hate Crimes against Disabled People." *Social Alternatives* 19, no. 4: 23–30.

———. 2003. "Disability Hate Crimes: More Common Than You Might Think." *Link* Magazine, August, 8–10.

Siebers, Tobin. 2002. "Broken Beauty: Disability and Art Vandalism." *Michigan Quarterly Review* 41, no. 2 (Spring): 223–45.

———. 2004. "Disability as Masquerade." *Literature and Medicine* 23, no. 1 (Spring): 1–22.

Sloan, Thomas G. N.d. "The Medical Supervision of School Children in South Manchester, Conn." New York: William Wood. Smith Ely Jelliffe Eugenics Collection.

Smart, Isabelle Thompson. 1913a. "The Physician and the Mentally Defective Child." Reprinted from *New York State Journal of Medicine*, June, 1–17. Read before the annual meeting of the New York State Medical Society, Albany, 29–30 April 1913. Smith Ely Jelliffe Eugenics Collection.

———. 1913b. "Studies in the Relation of Physical Inability and Mental Deficiency to the Body Social." Washington, D.C.: Government Printing Office. 8 pp. Reprinted from *Transactions of the Fifteenth International Congress of Hygiene and Demography, Held at Washington, D.C., September 23–28, 1912*. Smith Ely Jelliffe Eugenics Collection.

———. N.d. "The Mentally Defective Child—A Social Menace." 5 pp. Reprinted from *Proceedings of the Sixth Congress of the American School Hygiene Association*. Smith Ely Jelliffe Eugenics Collection.

Smart, Isabelle Thompson, and Mary Sutton Macy. 1911. "On the Medical Examination of Children Reported as Mentally Defective in the Public Schools." Reprinted from *Pediatrics* 23, no. 11 (11 November): 1–7. Smith Ely Jelliffe Eugenics Collection.

Smith, Adam. 1976a. *An Inquiry into the Nature of the Wealth of Nations*. Edited by R. H. Campbell, A. S. Skinner, and W. B. Todd. Oxford: Clarendon Press.

———. 1976b. *The Theory of Moral Sentiments*. Edited by D. D. Raphael and A. L. Macfie. Oxford: Oxford University Press.

Smith, Florence Givens. 1917. "Report on a Special Class of Eleven Defective Children." State Board of Charities: Mental Examinations, No. 9. *Eugenics and Social Welfare Bulletin* (Albany, N.Y.): 60–73. Smith Ely Jelliffe Eugenics Collection.

Smith, Stevenson, Madge W. Wilkinson, and Louisa C. Wagoner. 1914. "A Summary of the Laws of the Several States Governing: I. Marriage and Divorce of the Feebleminded, the Epileptic, and the Insane; II. Asexualization; III. Institutional Commitment and Discharge of the Feebleminded and Epileptic." Bulletin of the University of Washington, No. 82. The Bailey and Babette Gatzert Foundation for Child Welfare. 87 pp. Smith Ely Jelliffe Eugenics Collection.

Snyder, Sharon, and David Mitchell. 2002. "Out of the Ashes of Eugenics: United States Diagnostic Regimes and the Making of a Disability Minority." *Patterns of Prejudice* 36, no. 1: 79–103.

Sobchack, Vivian. 1991. *The Address of the Eye: A Phenomenology of Film Experience.* Princeton, N.J.: Princeton University Press.

Soloway, Richard A. 1990. *Demography and Degeneration: Eugenics and the Declining Birthrate in Twentieth-Century Britain.* Chapel Hill: University of North Carolina Press.

Spivak, Gayatri. 1988. "Can the Subaltern Speak?" In *Marxism and the Interpretation of Culture*, ed. C. Nelson and L. Grossberg, 271–313. Urbana: University of Illinois Press.

———. 1993. *Outside in the Teaching Machine.* New York: Routledge.

Stafford, Barbara Maria. 1995. *Body Criticism: Imaging the Unseen in Enlightenment Art and Medicine.* Cambridge, Mass.: MIT Press.

Stanley, Amy Dru. 1998. *From Bondage to Contract: Wage Labor, Marriage, and the Market in the Age of Slave Emancipation.* New York: Cambridge University Press.

Starobinski, Jean. 1997. *Largesse.* Translated by J. M. Todd. Chicago: University of Chicago Press.

State Board of Charities, Department of State and Alien Poor. 1917a. "Report of the Mental Examination of Certain Pupils in the Thomas Indian School, Iroquois, N.Y." State Board of Charities: Mental Examinations, No. 9. *Eugenics and Social Welfare Bulletin* (Albany, N.Y.): 37–42. Smith Ely Jelliffe Eugenics Collection.

State Board of Charities, Department of State and Alien Poor, Bureau of Analysis and Investigation. 1917b. "Mental Examinations." *Eugenics and Social Welfare Bulletin* (Albany, N.Y.), no. 11: 5–59. Smith Ely Jelliffe Eugenics Collection.

Stearns, A. Warren. 1916. "What Recent Investigations Have Shown to Be the Relation between Mental Defect and Crime." Boston: Massachusetts Society for Mental Hygiene. 6 pp. Reprinted from the *Boston Medical and Surgical Journal* 175, no. 12 (21 September): 400–408. Read at the conference of the Massachusetts Society for Mental Hygiene, Boston, 18 November 1915. Smith Ely Jelliffe Eugenics Collection.

Stevens, H. C. N.d. "The Causes of Feeblemindedness." Smith Ely Jelliffe Eugenics Collection.

Stevenson, George S. 1925. "The Physiology of the Feebleminded." Chicago: American Medical Association. 7 pp. Reprinted from *Archives of Neurology and Psychiatry* 13 (April): 497–503. Smith Ely Jelliffe Eugenics Collection.

Stewart, Susan. 1993. *On Longing: Narratives of the Miniature, the Gigantic, the Souvenir, the Collection.* Durham, N.C.: Duke University Press.

Stiker, Henri-Jacques. 1999. *A History of Disability.* Translated by W. Sayers. Ann Arbor: University of Michigan Press.

Stone, Deborah. 1984. *The Disabled State.* Philadelphia: Temple University Press.

Thomson, Rosemarie Garland. 1997. *Extraordinary Bodies: Figuring Physical Disability in American Culture and Literature.* New York: Columbia University Press.

Thoreau, Henry David. 1973. "Economy." In *Reform Papers*, ed. Wendell Glick. Princeton, N.J.: Princeton University Press.

———. 1998 [1863]. "Life without Principle." In *Civil Disobedience, Solitude, and Life without Principle.* Buffalo, N.Y.: Prometheus Books.

Trattner, Walter I. 1994. *From Poor Law to Welfare State: A History of Social Welfare in America.* 5th ed. New York: Basic Books.

Tredgold, A. F. 1917. "Moral Imbecility." *Practitioner* 39:43–56.

————. 1929. "The Relationship of Mental Deficiency to Mental Disease in General." *Mott Memorial Volume*, 107–24. Smith Ely Jelliffe Eugenics Collection.

Tremain, Shelley. 2002. "On the Subject of Impairment." In *Disability/Postmodernity: Embodying Disability Theory*, ed. M. Corker and T. Shakespeare, 32–47. London: Continuum.

Trent, James. 1994. *Inventing the Feeble Mind: A History of Mental Retardation in the United States*. Berkeley: University of California Press.

Trimp, Helen P. 1987. *Melville's Confidence Man and American Politics in the 1850s*. Hamden, Conn.: Archon Books.

Twenty-Sixth Annual Report of the Managers of the State Lunatic Asylum, For the Year 1868. Transmitted to the Legislature January 28, 1869. Albany, N.Y.: Argus Company, Printers. Smith Ely Jelliffe Eugenics Collection.

UPIAS. 1976. *Fundamental Principles of Disability*. London: Union of Physically Impaired Against Segregation. http://www.leeds.ac.uk/disability-studies/archiveuk/UPIAS/fundamental%20principles.pdf (accessed 22 June 2004).

Ventura, Michael. 1988. "Report from El Dorado." In *Multi Cultural Literacy*, ed. R. Simmonson and S. Walker, 173–88. St. Paul, Minn.: Graywolf Press.

Vogt, S. 2002. "Epistemologies of Eugenics: Gender and Resistance in Two Works of U.S. and German Literature." Master's thesis, University of Illinois at Chicago.

Wallin, J. E. W. 1920. "The Concept of the Feeble-Minded, Especially the Moron." *Training School Bulletin* 17, no. 3 (May; whole number 175): 41–53. Delivered, in substance, before Section H, Anthropology and Psychology, of the American Association for the Advancement of Science, 29 December 1920. Smith Ely Jelliffe Eugenics Collection.

Watkins, Daniel P. 1983. "The Ideological Dimensions of Byron's *The Deformed Transformed*." *Criticism* 25, no. 1 (Winter): 27–40.

Watkins, John. 1822. *Memoirs of the Life and Writings of Lord Byron*. London: H. Colburn.

Waugh, Joan. 2001. "'Give This Man Work!' Josephine Shaw Lowell, the Charity Organization Society of the City of New York, and the Depression of 1893." *Social Science History* 25, no. 2: 217–46.

Weindling, Paul. 1989. *Health, Race and German Politics between National Unification and Nazism, 1870–1945*. Cambridge: Cambridge University Press.

Wells, Frederic Lyman. 1916. "The Child Nation." *School and Society* 4, no. 91 (23 September): 486–87.

Wendell, Susan. 1996. *The Rejected Body: Feminist Philosophical Reflections on Disability*. New York: Routledge.

Westin, Alan. 1976. "'You Start Off with a Bromide': Wiseman on Film and Civil Liberties." In *Frederick Wiseman*, ed. Thomas R. Atkins. New York: Monarch.

Williams, Linda. 1999. "Film Bodies: Gender, Genre, and Excess." In *Film Theory and Criticism*, ed. Leo Braudy and Marshall Cohen, 701–15. Oxford: Oxford University Press.

Williams, Tom A. 1917. "Racial Factors of Delinquency." *Anthropology*. Paper presented before the Second Pan American Scientific Congress, Washington, D.C., 27 December 1915–8 January 1916. Washington, D.C.: Government Printing Office.

Wills, David. 1995. *Prosthesis*. Stanford, Calif.: Stanford University Press.

Winthrop, John. 1997. "A Modell of Christian Charity." In *The English Literatures of America: 1500–1800*, 151–59. New York: Routledge.

Wiseman, Frederick. *See under* "Films," *below*.

Wolbring, Gregor. 2000. "Science and the Disadvantaged." Edmonds Institute Occasional Papers, Edmonds, Wash.

Woodhull and Claflin's Weekly. 1871. http://www.victoria-woodhull.com/wcwarchive .htm.

Woolf, Virginia. 1928. *A Room of One's Own*. New York: Harvest Books.

Wright, Conrad Edick. 1992. *The Transformation of Charity in Postrevolutionary New England*. Boston: Northeastern University Press.

Yale, Caroline A. 1916. "A Plea for the Instruction and After-School Care of the Feeble-Minded Deaf." *Boston Medical and Surgical Journal* 177, no. 14 (4 October): 490–92. Read before the Conference on Feeble-mindedness of the Massachusetts Society for Mental Hygiene, Boston, 15 December 1916. Smith Ely Jelliffe Eugenics Collection.

Yeazell, Ruth Bernard. 1988. "Henry James." In *Columbia Literary History of the United States*, ed. Emory Elliott, 668–89. New York: Columbia University Press.

FILMS

Adjustment and Work. 1986. Directed by Frederick Wiseman. Zipporah Films.

Afraid of the Dark. 1991. Directed by Mark Peploe. Fine Line Pictures.

Animal House. 1978. Directed by John Landis. Universal Pictures.

Are You Fit to Marry? 1927. John E. Allen, Inc. (Also issued as *The Black Stork* [1917].)

Blind. 1987. Directed by Frederick Wiseman. Zipporah Films.

Crash. 1996. Directed by David Cronenberg. Fine Line Pictures.

Dark Victory. 1939. Directed by Edmund Goulding. Warner Bros.

Deaf. 1986. Directed by Frederick Wiseman. Zipporah Films.

Dumb and Dumberer: When Harry Met Lloyd. 2003. Directed by Troy Miller. New Line Cinema.

Even Dwarfs Started Small. 1970. Directed by Werner Herzog. Anchor Bay Entertainment.

Forbidden Maternity (Maternité Interdite). 2002. Directed by Diane Maroger. Athenaise Productions.

Forrest Gump. 1994. Directed by Robert Zemeckis. Paramount Studios.

Freaks. 1932. Directed by Tod Browning. MGM Films.

Gattaca. 1997. Directed by Andrew Niccol. Columbia.

Girl, Interrupted. 1999. Directed by James Mangold. Columbia Tristar.

Hannibal. 2001. Directed by Ridley Scott. MGM/Universal.

Hospital. 1970. Directed by Frederick Wiseman. Zipporah Films.

Jennifer 8. 1992. Directed by Bruce Robinson. Paramount Studios.

The Men. 1950. Directed by Fred Zinnemann. Republic Pictures.

Minority Report. 2002. Directed by Steven Spielberg. 20th Century Fox.

The Miracle Worker. 1962. Directed by Arthur Penn. MGM/UA.

Multi-handicapped. 1986. Directed by Frederick Wiseman. Zipporah Films.

One Flew over the Cuckoo's Nest. 1975. Directed by Milos Forman. Warner Studios.

Peeping Tom. 1960. Directed by Michael Powell. Astor.

Philadelphia. 1993. Directed by Jonathan Demme. Columbia Tristar Studios.

Rain Man. 1988. Directed by Barry Levinson. MGM.

Richard III. 1955. Directed by Laurence Olivier and Anthony Bushell. Lopert.

Richard III. 1995. Directed by Richard Loncraine. MGM/Universal Artists.

Self Preservation: The Art of Riva Lehrer. 2004. Directed by Sharon Snyder. Brace Yourselves Productions.

Silent Night, Deadly Night 3: Better Watch Out! 1989. Directed by Monte Hellman. Quiet.

Speed. 1994. Directed by Jan de Bont. 20th Century Fox.

Star Wars: Episode V—The Empire Strikes Back. 1980. Directed by Irvin Kershner. 20th Century Fox.

Stuck on You. 2003. Directed by Peter and Bobby Farrelly. 20th Century Fox.

Titicut Follies. 1967. Directed by Frederick Wiseman. Zipporah Films.

Touch of Evil. 1958. Directed by Orson Welles. Universal.

Unbreakable. 2000. Directed by M. Night Shyamalan. Buena Vista.

Vital Signs: Crip Culture Talks Back. 1995. Directed by Sharon Snyder. Brace Yourselves Productions.

Wait until Dark. 1967. Directed by Terence Young. Warner Bros.

When Billy Broke His Head. 1995. Directed by Billy Golfus. Independent Television Service.

A World without Bodies. 2002. Directed by Sharon Snyder. Brace Yourselves Productions.

X-Men. 2000. Directed by Bryan Singer. 20th Century Fox.

X2: X-Men United. 2003. Directed by Bryan Singer. 20th Century Fox.

INDEX